Type 2 Diabetes in 2026 - From Long History to Near Outlook

Edited by Rudolf Chlup

Published in London, United Kingdom

Type 2 Diabetes in 2026 - From Long History to Near Outlook
http://dx.doi.org/10.5772/intechopen.1005941
Edited by Rudolf Chlup

Contributors
Abdullah Ahmed, Ahmed Ahmed, Alexia Assaad, B. Kalpana Kosalram, Biayni Minasyan, Faisal Khalid A. Zakri, Fernando Grover Páez, Irene Sambath, Jaya Bhanu Kanwar, Jenna Al-Hammady, Luis Diego Pantoja Chong, Luz Elena Cortes Bautista, Olufunmilayo Moronwiyan, Samah Ismail, Serdar Serdar, Sofía Zubieta Barrios, V. Srinivas, Ximena Guadalupe Reynoso Velazquez

First published in London, United Kingdom, 2026 by IntechOpen
IntechOpen is the global imprint of INTECHOPEN LIMITED, registered in England and Wales, registration number: 11086078, 167-169 Great Portland Street, London, W1W 5PF, United Kingdom

For EU product safety concerns: IN TECH d.o.o., Prolaz Marije Krucifikse Kozulić 3, 51000 Rijeka, Croatia, info@intechopen.com or visit our website at intechopen.com.

British Library Cataloguing-in-Publication Data
A catalogue record for this book is available from the British Library

Type 2 Diabetes in 2026 - From Long History to Near Outlook
Edited by Rudolf Chlup
p. cm.
Print ISBN 978-1-83634-647-0
Online ISBN 978-1-83634-646-3
eBook (PDF) ISBN 978-1-83634-648-7

If disposing of this product, please recycle the paper responsibly.

Meet the editor

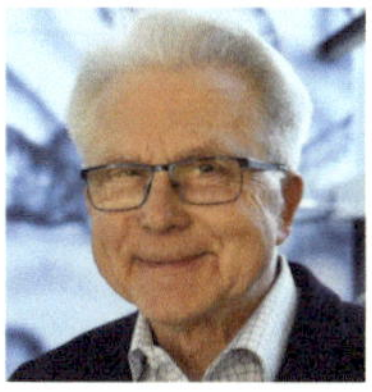

Rudolf Chlup graduated from Palacký University Olomouc, Czechia, and attended postgraduate courses in Prague, Karlsburg, Edinburgh, London, Bucharest, Moscow, Sophia, Düsseldorf, and San Francisco. He is a consultant in internal medicine and diabetology at the Teaching Hospital Olomouc, Czech Republic. He earned the title of Dr. Med. Habil. at the University of Greifswald, Germany, in 1993. He has been a Professor of Medicine at Palacký University Olomouc since 2020. His research interests include diabetes management, comprising diet, exercise, education, medication, and technology. He is a member of the Czech, German, European, and American Diabetes Associations, as well as the executive committee of the Diabetes Education Study Group of the European Association for the Study of Diabetes (DESG/EASD). In 2015, Dr. Chlup received the Rudolf Korec Award from the Slovakian Diabetes Association.

Contents

Preface

The medical, social, and cultural history of diabetes dates back approximately 1,500 years BC, when "a disease with excessive urinary output" was described, as stated in the Ebers Papyrus, discovered in Egypt in the 19th century. The name "diabetes" was used as late as 200 BC by Demetrios of Apamaia. Further important historical milestones, including key discoveries like insulin, gliflozins, incretin preparations and recent technical equipment like glucometers, subcutaneous sensors, insulin pumps, etc., have already been referenced in literature focused on diabetes, which is available in libraries all over the world and also in websites, e.g.

- Engelhardt D. Diabetes: Its medical and cultural history. Springer Verlag Berlin-Heidelberg, 1989. Pages 491.

- Jörgens V. Die Geschichte der Diabetesforschung. Vom Opium zum Insulin. (The history of diabetes research. From Opium to Insulin.German). Auflage (Edition) 1, 2022. Verlag (Published in) Kirchheim, Mainz, 303 Seiten (Pages).

- Pantea Stoian A, editor. Type 2 Diabetes - From Pathophysiology to Cyber Systems [Internet]. IntechOpen; 2021. Available from: http://dx.doi.org/10.5772/intechopen.87312.

- Chlup R, editor. Type 2 Diabetes in 2024 - From Early Suspicion to Effective Management [Internet]. IntechOpen; 2023. Available from: http://dx.doi.org/10.5772/intechopen.1000405.

This book provides a short overview of the professional management of type 2 diabetes (T2D). The purpose of this edition is to support healthcare professionals and students of general medicine in transferring recent knowledge to routine diabetes practice.

The book comprises six chapters, organized into two sections. The first section deals with the assessment of therapeutic effectiveness on diabetes and includes two chapters:

1. Anthropometric Measures and Type 2 Diabetes: Evaluating Predictors for Risk and Management

2. Assessment of Personal Glucometers for Routine Monitoring

The second section focuses on the management of type 2 diabetes and its complications. It includes four chapters:

1. Exercise and Type 2 Diabetes Mellitus

2. New and Interesting Benefits with New Molecules in Obesity and Type 2 Diabetes

3. Lived Experience of Diabetes Self-Management among the Elderly in India

4. Sarcopenia and Type 2 Diabetes Mellitus: Evaluation, Pathophysiological Links, and Management Strategies

Written by specialists in diabetes from various Institutions in different countries, including the Czech Republic, Egypt, India, the Kingdom of Saudi Arabia, and Mexico.

With its comprehensive coverage, this volume serves as a valuable resource for family physicians, diabetologists, educators, nurses, students, and other interested readers.

I want to thank the staff at IntechOpen, especially Author Service Manager Ms. Laura Divic, for her continuous assistance throughout the publication process.

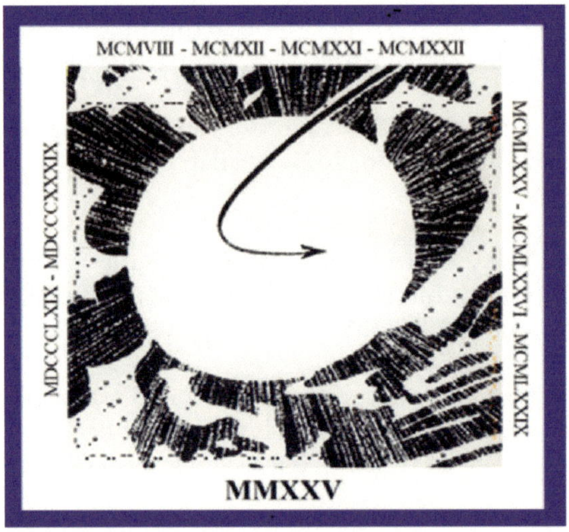

Mission: from recent history to dawning future (years of milestones in diabetes management). Roman numerals at figure margins serve as reminders of important dates related to pancreas function [1, 2], insulin implementation to human medicine [3], technology for insulin substitution and supplementation [4–8], therapeutic exercise [9], risk of atherosclerosis [10], trials on experimental diabetes in the rat [11], and implementation of incretins to type 2 management [12], all of which created a base for the topics presented in this book [13].

Rudolf Chlup
2nd Department of Medicine, Gastroenterology and Geriatrics,
Teaching Hospital Olomouc,
Olomouc, Czech Republic

Department of Diabetes Moravský Beroun Institute of Specialized Treatments
Paseka,
Paseka, Czech Republic

Department of Physiology,
Faculty of Medicine and Dentistry,
Palacký University Olomouc,
Olomouc, Czech Republic

References

[1] Langerhans P. Beiträge zur mikroscopischen Anatomie der Bauchspeicheldrüse. (Contributions to microscopic anatomy of Pancreas. German.) Wilhelms-Friedrich Wilhelm Universität zu Berlin, printed by G. Lange; 1869

[2] Mering J, Minkowski O. Diabetes mellitus nach Pankreas extirpation. (Diabetes mellitus following the pancreatectomy. German.). Zbl Klin Med. 1889;**10**:393-394

[3] Banting FG, Best CH. Pancreatic extracts. Journal of Laboratory and Clinical Medicine. May 22;7(8):3-11

[4] Pickup JC, Keen H, Parsons JS, et al. Continuous subcutaneous insulin infusion: an approach to achieving normoglycaemia. British Medical Journal. 1978;**282**:347-350

[5] Paton JS, Wilson M, Ireland JT, Reith SB. Convenient pocket insulin syringe. The Lancet. 1981;**317**(8213):189-190

[6] Janů K, Chlup R, Chleboun J. Ruční mechanický dávkovač kapaliny Úřad pro patenty a objevy v Praze: Číslo žádosti PV 6160, podaná dne 24. 8. 1983, číslo patentu 237521, datum udělení patentu 24. 4. 1985. (Manual mechanical device for fluid dosing. Patent and Inventions Office Prague: Application number PV 6160 submitted on 24. 8. 1983, Patent number 237521, was granted by the patent office on 24. 4. 1985. Czech.)

[7] Rex J, Vogeley OA. Dispenser. U.S.patent number 4,592,745 [Application Number 06/584,876], submitted on 1984-02-29, was granted by the patent office on 1986-06-03

[8] Berger M, Jörgens V, Mühlhauser I. Rationale for the use of insulin therapy alone as the pharmacological treatment of type 2 diabetes. Diabetes Care 1999;**22**(Suppl 3):C71-C75

[9] Koivisto VA, Shervin RS. Exercise in diabetes. Therapeutic implications. Postgraduate Medicine 1979;**66**:87

[10] Stout RW. Diabetes and atherosclerosis – the role of insulin. Diabetologie 1979;**16**:14110

[11] Korec R. Experimental and spontaneous diabetes mellitus in the rat and mouse. Edition Center of University PJ Šafárik, Košice, ČSFR, Košice. 1991. pp. 1-246

[12] Bruns W, Fiedler H, Altman B, Lundershausen R, Menzel R, Worms F, et al. Insulintherapie bei Typ 2 Diabetes Pathophysiologisch begründete Therapie mit Insulin unter besonderer Berücksichtigung der Insulinresistenz und des Inkretineffektes. (Insulin treatment in T2D Pathophysiology-based insulin treatment with particular consideration of insulin resistance and incretins. German.) 2. Auflage; UNIMED Verlag, AG, Bremen, 2010

[13] Type 2 Diabetes in 2024 – From Early Suspicion to Effective Management. London, UK: IntechOpen; 2024

Section 1

Assessment of Therapeutic Effectiveness on Diabetes

Chapter 1

Anthropometric Measures and Type 2 Diabetes: Evaluating Predictors for Risk and Management

Faisal Khalid A. Zakri

Abstract

Anthropometric indices are vital in evaluating obesity, a key factor in developing type 2 diabetes mellitus (T2DM). This chapter reviews the effectiveness of measures like body mass index (BMI), waist circumference (WC), waist-to-hip ratio (WHR), and body shape index (ABSI) in predicting diabetes risks. This chapter emphasizes the importance of tailored thresholds for different populations by focusing on Saudi Arabia's and global studies' findings. Emerging tools, including waist-to-height ratio (WHtR), are explored alongside advanced technologies such as artificial intelligence and 3D body imaging to enhance risk assessment and diabetes management. Anthropometric measures are indispensable for evaluating obesity, a key risk factor for type 2 diabetes mellitus (T2DM). This chapter examines the predictive value of indices such as body mass index (BMI), waist circumference (WC), waist-to-hip ratio (WHR), and body shape index (ABSI). Leveraging findings from Saudi populations and global systematic reviews, it highlights population-specific thresholds and the role of central adiposity in disease progression. Emerging metrics like ABSI and waist-to-height ratio (WHtR) are evaluated alongside traditional measures. The chapter also discusses integrating advanced technologies, including artificial intelligence (AI) and 3D imaging, to enhance diabetes risk prediction.

Keywords: anthropometric measures, type 2 diabetes, a body shape index, waist circumference, risk stratification

1. Introduction

Note: The term 'body mass' is used in this chapter to reflect scientific precision, though it is often referred to as 'weight' in non-technical contexts.

Type 2 diabetes mellitus (T2DM) is a growing global concern, with projections estimating a significant increase in prevalence by 2045. Obesity, particularly central obesity, is strongly associated with the development of insulin resistance and T2DM. Due to their simplicity and cost-effectiveness, anthropometric measures, such as BMI, WC, and WHR, are widely utilized for assessing obesity-related health risks. However, these indices have limitations, leading to the development of alternative metrics like ABSI and WHtR. This chapter examines the significance of these measures in predicting diabetes risks and highlights technological advancements for improving their accuracy and utility.

Type 2 diabetes mellitus (T2DM) represents a significant global health challenge, with its prevalence projected to increase from 463 million in 2019 to 700 million by 2045 [1]. Obesity, particularly central obesity, is a primary driver of T2DM due to its association with insulin resistance, chronic inflammation, and metabolic dysregulation [2]. Anthropometric measures such as BMI, WC, and WHR provide simple, cost-effective tools to assess obesity-related risks. This chapter explores these measures' relevance, utility, and limitations, focusing on population-specific findings and their integration with advanced technologies.

2. Anthropometric indices

2.1 Body mass index (BMI)

BMI is one of the most commonly used metrics for classifying individuals based on their body mass relative to height. Although widely adopted, BMI fails to distinguish between fat and lean mass, limiting its accuracy in assessing central obesity—a key factor in T2DM risk. Despite these limitations, BMI remains a valuable tool for population-level obesity monitoring.

BMI is the most commonly used anthropometric measure for categorizing individuals as underbody mass, normal body mass, overbody mass, or obese. It is calculated using the formula:

$$BMI = \text{weight}\left(kg\right) / \text{height}\left(\text{m}\right) \hat{} 2 \qquad (1)$$

Although widely utilized, BMI has limitations as it does not differentiate between lean and fat mass. Studies indicate that BMI is a better indicator of general obesity than central adiposity, which is more closely associated with T2DM risk [3].

2.2 Waist circumference (WC) and waist-to-hip ratio (WHR)

WC and WHR are critical measures for assessing fat distribution, which is more directly linked to metabolic disorders like T2DM. These indices outperform BMI in predicting central obesity-related risks. For instance, WC thresholds of >102 cm for men and > 88 cm for women are widely accepted, while WHR thresholds are 0.90 for men and 0.85 for women. These metrics provide a more targeted assessment of central adiposity.

WC and WHR are superior to BMI in predicting central obesity and its related complications, including T2DM. WHO guidelines define abdominal obesity as WC >102 cm for men and > 88 cm for women, while WHR thresholds are 0.90 for men and 0.85 for women [4]. These measures account for fat distribution, providing a better assessment of metabolic risk.

2.3 A body shape index (ABSI)

ABSI is a relatively new metric that adjusts WC for height and body mass, offering a more precise measure of central obesity. Unlike traditional indices, ABSI has been shown to correlate strongly with mortality risk and metabolic complications, making it a valuable tool for identifying high-risk individuals.

ABSI, introduced in 2012, adjusts WC for height and body mass to provide a more nuanced measure of central obesity. It is calculated as follows:

$$\text{ABSI} = WC / \left(BMI \wedge (2/3) \times \text{height} \wedge (1/2) \right) \tag{2}$$

Research suggests that ABSI correlates more strongly with all-cause mortality and T2DM risk than traditional measures like BMI and WC [5]. This index offers the potential for identifying high-risk individuals whom conventional metrics might overlook.

2.4 Waist-to-height ratio (WHtR)

WHtR is an emerging metric that uses the waist circumference to height ratio to assess obesity-related risks. With a universal cutoff of 0.5, WHtR is less influenced by population-specific variability, making it a promising alternative to other indices.

WHtR has emerged as a simple and effective measure for assessing central obesity. Unlike WC and WHR, WHtR accounts for height, making it less susceptible to population-specific variability. A WHtR cutoff of 0.5 is commonly recommended for identifying individuals at risk of T2DM and cardiovascular diseases [6].

3. Findings from Saudi Arabian cohorts

The relationship between anthropometric indices and diabetes risk varies across populations due to genetic, environmental, and lifestyle differences. **Table 1** presents comparative BMI, WC, WHR, and ABSI data for Saudi Arabia and the USA. While the USA exhibits higher levels of central obesity, as indicated by larger WC and WHR values, ABSI remains relatively consistent across populations, suggesting its potential as a universal index. These findings emphasize the importance of tailoring obesity thresholds to specific populations for more accurate risk assessment.

Research in Saudi Arabia reinforces the significance of anthropometric indices in predicting T2DM risks. A 2019 study of 120 adults found that ABSI was more effective than BMI in identifying individuals with high central adiposity, particularly those with normal or below-average BMI. This underscores the need for population-specific

Country	BMI (mean ± SD)	WC (cm)	WHR	ABSI
Saudi Arabia	27.5 ± 3.2	98.3 ± 4.1	0.91	0.08
USA	29.1 ± 4.5	102.5 ± 5.0	0.95	0.09

Table 1.
Comparative epidemiological data for anthropometric measures.

thresholds and interventions to improve diabetes risk prediction and management [7]. These findings underscore the importance of population-specific thresholds and the need for tailored interventions.

4. Comparative insights from systematic reviews

The prevalence of type 2 diabetes mellitus (T2DM) and obesity-related anthropometric indicators varies significantly across regions, reflecting differences in body composition and risk factors. **Table 2** provides an overview of these prevalences and mean values for BMI, WC, WHR, and ABSI across selected countries. The data highlight that while obesity prevalence is high in developed nations like the USA, countries such as Saudi Arabia show similar trends in central obesity and T2DM prevalence. These patterns underscore the global challenge of diabetes and the importance of adopting context-specific anthropometric measures for effective risk assessment and early diagnosis.

Systematic reviews and meta-analyses further emphasize that WC and WHR outperform BMI predicting T2DM and its complications. Additionally, ABSI offers enhanced predictive value, particularly in diverse populations where body composition varies widely.

4.1 Meta-analyses on anthropometric predictors

Global meta-analyses consistently demonstrate the superiority of WC and WHR over BMI in predicting T2DM and its complications. For instance, a 2021 analysis reported that WC and WHR were stronger predictors of insulin resistance and cardiovascular risk than BMI [8].

5. Challenges and future directions

5.1 Limitations of current measures

While traditional anthropometric measures such as body mass index (BMI) and waist circumference (WC) remain valuable for assessing obesity-related risks, they have notable limitations. BMI does not differentiate between fat and muscle mass, while WC lacks standardized thresholds across different ethnic groups. These limitations underscore the need for alternative metrics to provide more precise and universally applicable assessments.

Emerging indices like waist-to-height ratio (WHtR) and A body shape index (ABSI) address some of these shortcomings. WHtR, with its universal cutoff of 0.5,

Country	Prevalence of T2DM (%)	Obesity prevalence (%)	BMI (mean ± SD)	WC (cm)	WHR	ABSI
Saudi Arabia	18.3	35.4	27.5 ± 3.2	98.3 ± 4.1	0.91	0.08
USA	11.3	42.4	29.1 ± 4.5	102.5 ± 5.0	0.95	0.09
India	8.9	18.7	23.2 ± 2.8	91.4 ± 3.8	0.87	0.07

Table 2.
Prevalence of type 2 diabetes and obesity indicators by country.

Metric	Formula	Cutoff value	Predictive accuracy	Limitation
BMI	Weight (kg)/height (m)^2	≥25	Moderate	Does not account for fat distribution
WHR	Waist circumference/hip circumference	Men: ≥0.90, women: ≥0.85	High	Population-specific variability
WHtR	Waist circumference/height	Universal: ≥0.5	High	Requires validation in large cohorts
ABSI	WC/(BMI^(2/3) × height^(1/2))	—	Strong correlation with mortality risk	Complex formula

Table 3.
Emerging anthropometric metrics in risk prediction.

reduces the need for population-specific adjustments, making it a promising tool for global use. ABSI incorporates WC, height, and body mass into its calculation, offering insights into central obesity and mortality risk. **Table 3** summarizes these emerging metrics, their formulas, cutoff values, and predictive capabilities compared to traditional measures.

Despite their potential, these indices require further validation across diverse populations to ensure accuracy and reliability in different contexts. Integrating WHtR and ABSI into clinical practice could bridge gaps left by traditional metrics, enabling more precise assessments of central obesity and its role in metabolic disorders like type 2 diabetes mellitus (T2DM) [9].

5.2 Emerging technologies

Advanced technologies such as 3D body imaging and AI-driven predictive models are transforming the landscape of anthropometric assessments. These tools provide precise body composition measurements and enable personalized risk assessments for T2DM. However, challenges related to cost, accessibility, and integration into clinical practice remain.

Advancements in 3D body scanning and AI-based analytics are revolutionizing anthropometric assessments. These technologies enable precise body composition measurements, offering personalized risk profiles for T2DM. However, challenges such as cost, accessibility, and integration into clinical workflows remain [10].

6. Conclusion

Anthropometric indices remain essential tools for evaluating obesity-related risks of T2DM. While traditional measures like BMI and WC are valuable, emerging tools such as ABSI and WHtR offer enhanced predictive capabilities. Integrating these measures with advanced technologies will improve their utility in clinical and public health settings.

Anthropometric measures remain essential tools for assessing obesity-related T2DM risks. Traditional metrics like BMI and WC and emerging indices like ABSI and WHtR provide a comprehensive framework for evaluating central adiposity. Integrating advanced technologies will enhance their utility in clinical and public health settings.

Author details

Faisal Khalid A. Zakri
Diabetes and Family Medicine Consultant, Ministry of Health,
Kingdom of Saudi Arabia

*Address all correspondence to: faisal.zakri11@gmail.com

References

[1] Aschner P, Karuranga S, James S, Simmons D, Basit A, Shaw JE, et al. The International Diabetes Federation's guide for diabetes epidemiological studies. Diabetes Research and Clinical Practice. 2021;**172**:108630. DOI: 10.1016/j.diabres.2020.108630

[2] Zimmet PZ, Alberti KGMM, Shaw J. Global and societal implications of the diabetes epidemic. Nature. 2001;**414**:782-787. DOI: 10.1038/414782a

[3] Nuttall FQ. Body mass index. Nutrition Today. 2015;**50**:117-128. DOI: 10.1097/NT.0000000000000092

[4] World Health Organisation (WHO). Waist Circumference and Waist–Hip Ratio. Report of a WHO Expert Consultation. Geneva; 2008. pp. 8-11

[5] Krakauer NY, Krakauer JC. A new body shape index predicts mortality hazard independently of body mass index. PLoS One. 2012;**7**(7):e39504. DOI: 10.1371/journal.pone.0039504

[6] Yoo E-G. Waist-to-height ratio as a screening tool for obesity and cardiometabolic risk. Korean Journal of Pediatrics. 2016;**59**:425. DOI: 10.3345/kjp.2016.59.11.425

[7] Saeed AA, Al-Hamdan NA. Anthropometric risk factors and predictors of hypertension among Saudi adult population – A national survey. Journal of Epidemiology and Global Health. 2013;**3**:197. DOI: 10.1016/j.jegh.2013.08.004

[8] Jayedi A, Soltani S, Motlagh SZ, Emadi A, Shahinfar H, Moosavi H, et al. Anthropometric and adiposity indicators and risk of type 2 diabetes: Systematic review and dose-response meta-analysis of cohort studies. BMJ. 2022:e067516. DOI: 10.1136/bmj-2021-067516

[9] Navya N, Udayakiran N. A comparative study of anthropometric measurements of children attending Urban and Rural Anganwadi Centres of a coastal district in Karnataka, India. International Journal of Community Medicine and Public Health. 2016;**4**;91. DOI: 10.18203/2394-6040.ijcmph20164717

[10] Bays HE, Fitch A, Cuda S, Gonsahn-Bollie S, Rickey E, Hablutzel J, et al. Artificial intelligence and obesity management: An Obesity Medicine Association (OMA) clinical practice statement (CPS) 2023. Obesity Pillars. 2023;**6**:100065. DOI: 10.1016/j.obpill.2023.100065

Chapter 2

Assessment of Personal Glucometers for Routine Monitoring

Biayni Minasyan, Jenna Al-Hammady, Abdullah Ahmed, Alexia Assaad, Serdar Serdar and Olufunmilayo Moronwiyan

Abstract

The purpose of this chapter is (1) to assess the accuracy and precision of two glucometer-strip systems (GSS): Galileo Glu/Ket (Wellion) and Newton GDH-FAD (Wellion), (2) to evaluate the relation between body mass index and glycemic response (BMI), and (3) to evaluate the effect of glycemic load (GL) on glycemic response. Capillary plasma glucose (cPG) measurement with a GSS determines the glycemic response. This study was performed within 6 months; with 10 volunteers, cPG was measured during three different one-hour sessions at ten-minute intervals, for each volunteer with the two evaluated GSS systems and a reference GSS system (Contour Plus One). The cPG values measured ranged between 2.9 and 9.3 mmol/L. Precision ranked as 1. Contour, 2. Newton, 3. Galileo. Contour Plus One showed the lowest variability. No significant difference in accuracy was shown between Galileo and Newton when compared to Contour reference. The control study provided similar results. Duration till maximum cPG achieved after ingestion of the glucose jelly was influenced by the glucose load; a higher glucose load takes longer to reach its maximum cPG values and return to baseline. The participants with a higher BMI had less effective glycemic responses with higher recorded cPG levels upon ingestion of a larger amount of GL during the study.

Keywords: GSS, cPG, Contour Plus One, Newton GDH-FAD (Wellion), Galileo Glu/Ket (Wellion), accuracy, precision, BMI, glycemic load, glycemic response, control study

1. Introduction

Ames Reflectance Meter, the first-ever blood glucose meter, was launched in 1970 by Miles Laboratories. It was bulky, expensive, and intended for hospital use only. Then, Anton H. Clemens invented the first portable glucose meter, the Ames Eyetone, paving the way for at-home blood sugar monitoring. However, it was not widely available to the public yet. Later, in 1981, Lifescan, a division of Johnson & Johnson, released the OneTouch meter, one of the first affordable and user-friendly devices to use at home. This was revolutionary, people with diabetes could finally monitor their blood glucose at home, in just seconds. More importantly, studies proved that frequent glucose monitoring dramatically reduces the risk of diabetes-related complications such as neuropathy, retinopathy, and nephropathy [1]. Today, glucometers are widely used, with digital displays, faster results, memory storage to track previous readings, and many more features to aid the user. They have become lifelines for millions, facilitating making daily decisions related to food, exercise, insulin, and safety. Modern glucometers have made the shift from reporting whole blood glucose to plasma-equivalent glucose to align with laboratory standards, which use plasma for testing. Plasma glucose levels are slightly higher than whole blood levels, so this change improves accuracy and consistency across home and clinical settings [2]. The international standard, ISO 15197:2013, specifies the requirements for *in vitro* glucose monitoring systems that measure glucose concentrations in capillary blood samples, and emphasizes the importance of plasma-equivalent reporting for consistency with laboratory results [3]. Glucometers still use capillary blood but convert the result to a plasma-equivalent value using a built-in software, to ensure results match lab readings and follow medical guidelines [4]. To measure the plasma glucose, glucometers generally use one of two enzyme systems: glucose oxidase or glucose dehydrogenase. Glucose oxidase system measures glucose by reacting with oxygen, producing hydrogen peroxide; it is glucose-specific but oxygen-dependent. On the other hand, the glucose dehydrogenase (GDH) System measures glucose *via* electron transfer using coenzymes such as PQQ and FAD; it is oxygen-independent but some types may lack glucose specificity. This raises the central question: which enzymatic system provides more accurate and precise glucose readings? [5]. In this study, two ISO-accredited GSS from Wellion, Galileo, which uses the glucose oxidase (Glu/Ket) method [6], and Newton, which employs the glucose dehydrogenase (GDH-FAD) method, were compared. The aim was to evaluate whether one outperforms the other in clinical accuracy. According to ISO 15197:2013, system accuracy is defined by the range within which 95% of the measured glucose values fall in comparison to a reference method, providing a standardized benchmark for performance assessment. The criteria states that 95% of the measured glucose values shall fall within either ±0.83 mmol/l (±15 mg/dl) of the average measured values of the reference measurement procedure at glucose concentrations <5.55 mmol/l (<100 mg/dl) or within ±15% at glucose concentrations ≥5.55 mmol/l (≥100 mg/dl) [7].

Contour Plus One, a third GSS, was used as the reference monitoring system. This was done because the Contour Plus One, which uses the glucose dehydrogenase (GDH-FAD) enzyme system itself, not only meets but exceeds the accuracy requirements [8, 9]. During user performance evaluations, Contour Plus One demonstrated high accuracy levels, with 97.7% of subject-obtained fingertip results and 100% of trial staff-obtained fingertip results [8]. Moreover, to assess further possible questions in this setting, the study additionally looks at the effect of factors like glycemic load and body mass index (BMI) on individual glycemic responses. The glycemic load (GL) measures the blood glucose elevating effect within food while glycemic index (GI) measures the speed of this effect. Foods with elevated glycemic load values generate more substantial blood glucose reactions [10]. Research shows that people with elevated BMI experience intensified blood glucose reactions after consuming meals with high GL values [11]. Hence, using cPG values within the range of 2.9–9.3 mmol/L, the study focused on the following questions (1) how do two commercial glucometers: Galileo Glu/Ket (Wellion) and Newton GDH-FAD (Wellion), perform with relation to their precision and accuracy, (2) how BMI affects individual glycemic responses, and (3) how glycemic loads affect glycemic responses.

2. Method

2.1 Scheduling, volunteers, and their characteristics

This trial was conducted between November 24, 2023, and April 16, 2024. A total of 10 volunteers (aged 19–34 years; BMI range: 18–31 kg/m^2) participated in three scheduled visits. Participants were required to fast (excluding water) for a minimum of 5 hours prior to each session. The cohort included two men and eight women; among them, one female volunteer reported daily use of e-cigarettes (three to four times per day). Eight volunteers engaged in regular physical activity, averaging two to three exercise sessions per week. None of the participants had a history or diagnosis of cardiovascular, pulmonary, autoimmune, or pancreatic diseases, including any form of diabetes mellitus.

2.2 Analytical and laboratory equipment

Three glucose self-monitoring systems (GSS) and up to three LOTs of test strips were utilized in this study. A total of 210 capillary plasma glucose (cPG) triplets were collected using the following devices: (1) Galileo Glu/Ket (Wellion), employing glucose oxidase-based strips; (2) Newton GDH-FAD (Wellion); and (3) Contour Plus One (Ascensia), utilizing glucose dehydrogenase-based strips (**Figures 1** and **2**). The accuracy of the Galileo and Newton devices was evaluated by comparing 630 corresponding results obtained from the Contour Plus One device, which is validated against the certified hexokinase-based analyzer, Cobas Integra 400. Measurement precision was assessed *via* the standard deviation (SD) of average differences within each of the 210 cPG triplets.

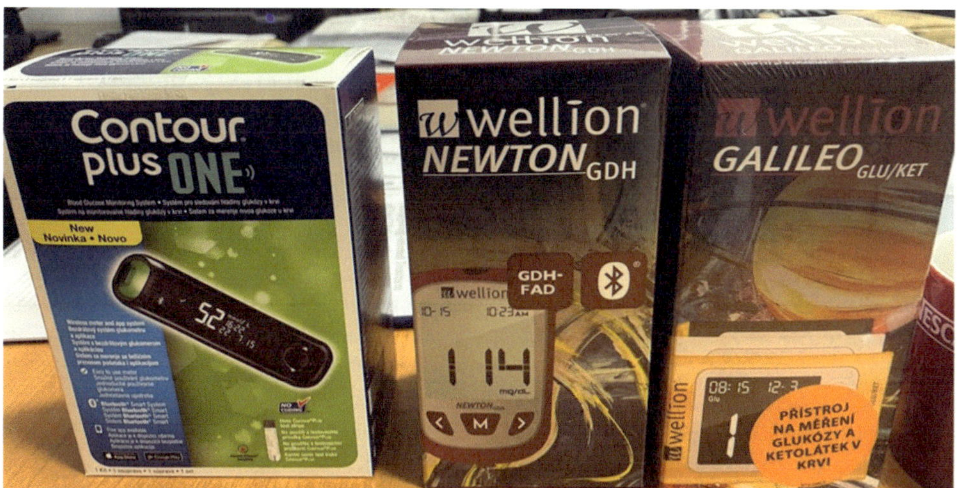

Figure 1.
The three GSS used: Contour Plus One (left), Newton GDH-FAD (middle), Galileo Glu/Ket (right).

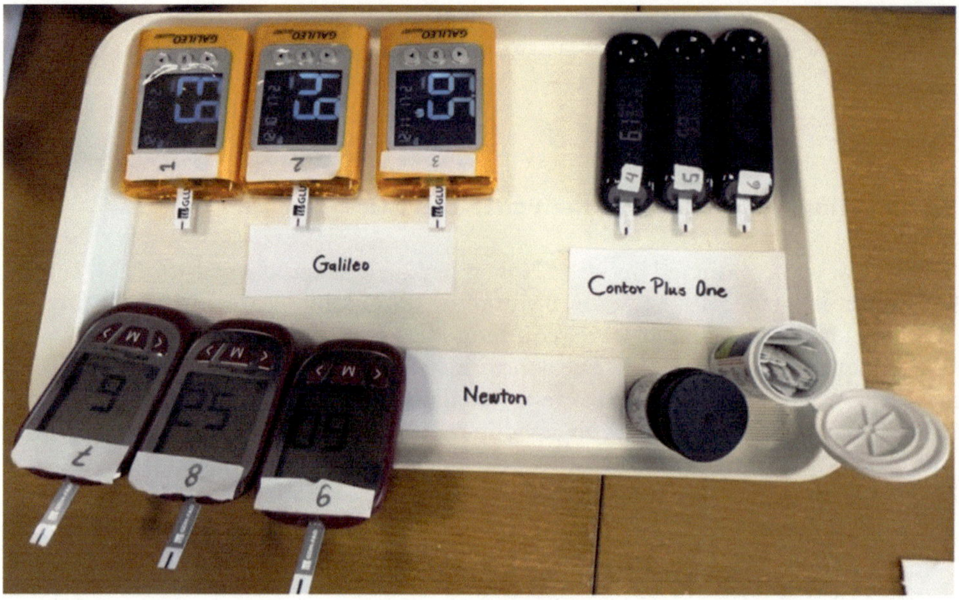

Figure 2.
The three GSS used: Contour Plus One (top right), Newton GDH-FAD (bottom), Galileo Glu/Ket (top left). All nine glucometers showing different values of cPG in mmol/L estimated from the same drop of blood collected from a single finger-prick.

Glycemic responses were induced using jelly-based GL containing 15 and 40 g of sucrose-fructose-glucose combinations (**Figure 3**), respectively, with both being produced by the Wellion brand. Each volunteer underwent the procedure mentioned below (see Section 2.3) three times on different days throughout the 6-month study period. The first day was with 15 g jelly, then with 40 g jelly, and lastly without administration of any sort of glucose load.

BMI was determined using a mechanical column scale, while height was confirmed verbally by each participant. The mean cPG values for the 15 and 40 g jelly groups were compared to the control values. Additionally, a Wilcoxon paired test was conducted to determine whether the glycemic loads of the two jelly amounts differed significantly.

Data analysis was performed using IBM SPSS Statistics for Windows, Version 23.0, with statistical significance set at $p < 0.05$.

2.3 Study design and data collection procedure

The study procedure followed a structured protocol described below, which was also illustrated as a video to demonstrate the process (see Video 1, https://intech-files.s3.amazonaws.com/a04Tc0000084zLMIAY/a09Tc000002fepxIAA/Videos%20%28Full%20Chapter%29-Assessment%20of%20personal%20glucometers%20for%20routine%20mon%20%282025-05-12%2014%3A29%3A24%29.zip).

Participants underwent standardized testing at each visit, following consistent pre-test conditions and device use across sessions to ensure the repeatability and reliability of the data. The procedure followed this subsequent order:

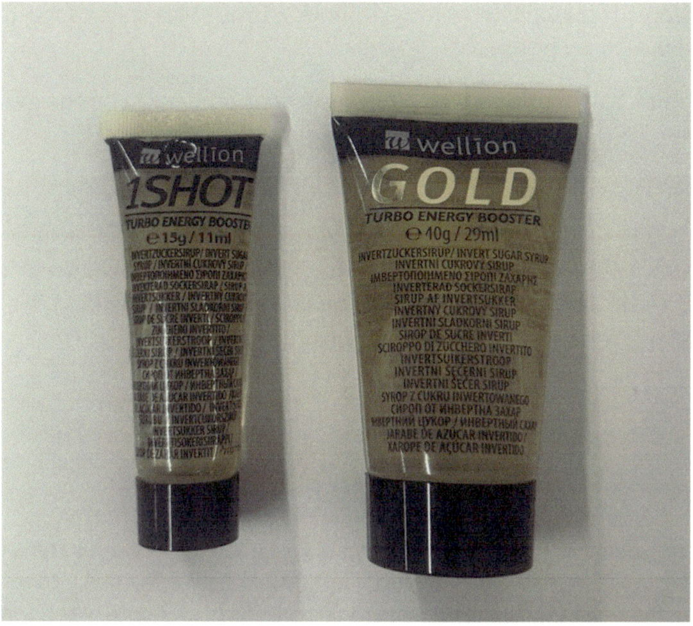

Figure 3.
Display of the 15 gram (left) and 40 gram (right) sucrose-fructose-glucose combination instant energy shots. Both contain vanilla flavored invert sugar syrup, with respective 54 and 144 kcal content [12, 13].

1. Patients arrived after having fasted for a minimum of 8 hours prior to the procedure to ensure a fasting state with the exclusion of water.

2. Fasting cPG levels were measured.

3. On two separate days, patients were administered a glucose-containing jelly, 15 g on the first day and 40 g on the next.

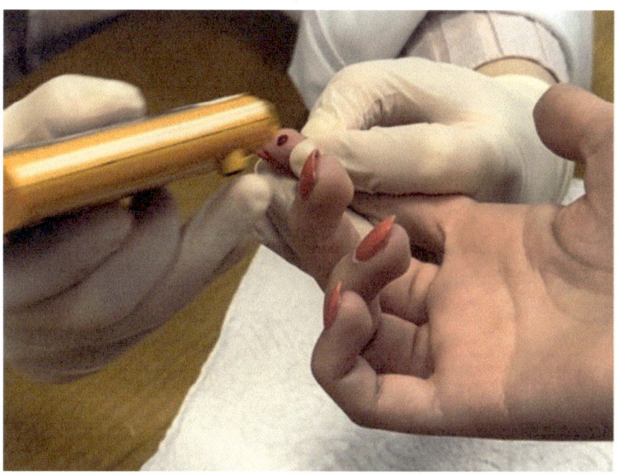

Figure 4.
The process of measuring cPG from a single finger-prick with one of the nine glucometers in action.

4. Immediately after the jelly was swallowed, a timer was started to monitor the time-dependent response.

5. From a single finger-prick, the cPG was measured using all nine glucometers (**Figure 4**).

6. At 10-minute intervals over the course of 1 hour, the same procedure was repeated under the same controlled conditions to assess glucose response over time.

Later, a control study was performed using an identical procedure with the single exception of no jelly being administered. The control study involved the same group of 10 volunteers.

3. Results

3.1 Impact of glucose load on glycemic response

Based on the Data Collection procedure at (2.3), the cPG values for each of the GSS systems (1. Galileo, 2. Contour Plus One, and 3. Newton) were recorded. Mean cPG values were calculated to standard deviation (**Table 1**), and values were further graphed (**Figures 5–7**).

GSS System_Time [min]	No glucose [mmol/l]		15 g glucose [mmol/l]		40 g glucose [mmol/l]	
	Mean	Standard deviation	Mean	Standard deviation	Mean	Standard deviation
Galileo_0	5.23	0.56	4.96	0.47	5.05	0.70
Contour_0	4.97	0.66	4.84	0.57	4.86	0.82
Newton_0	4.95	0.58	4.79	0.65	4.88	0.70
Galileo_10	5.05	0.52	5.00	0.47	5.47	0.77
Contour_10	4.91	0.69	4.92	0.69	5.40	0.77
Newton_10	4.86	0.63	4.96	0.63	5.41	0.71
Galileo_20	5.09	0.59	5.63	0.66	6.59	1.01
Contour_20	4.85	0.70	5.73	0.60	6.96	1.17
Newton_20	4.90	0.59	5.56	0.41	7.04	1.30
Galileo_30	5.13	0.50	5.50	0.72	7.21	1.21
Contour_30	4.99	0.52	5.51	0.63	7.28	1.23
Newton_30	5.02	0.65	5.40	0.66	7.03	1.34
Galileo_40	5.10	0.50	5.24	0.54	6.75	1.12
Contour_40	4.86	0.48	5.20	0.50	6.93	1.05
Newton_40	4.92	0.60	5.17	0.46	6.77	1.03
Galileo_50	4.99	0.51	4.92	0.44	6.26	1.14
Contour_50	4.76	0.57	4.93	0.43	6.33	1.24
Newton_50	4.72	0.60	4.81	0.41	6.19	1.16
Galileo_60	5.09	0.55	4.88	0.36	5.81	1.05
Contour_60	4.85	0.39	4.75	0.37	5.83	1.05
Newton_60	4.75	0.38	4.69	0.36	5.70	0.87

Table 1.
Mean cPG values with SD for the three GSS systems at each session, cPG reading was taken at a 10-minute interval, and each session was done on a separate day while the volunteers were in a fasted state.

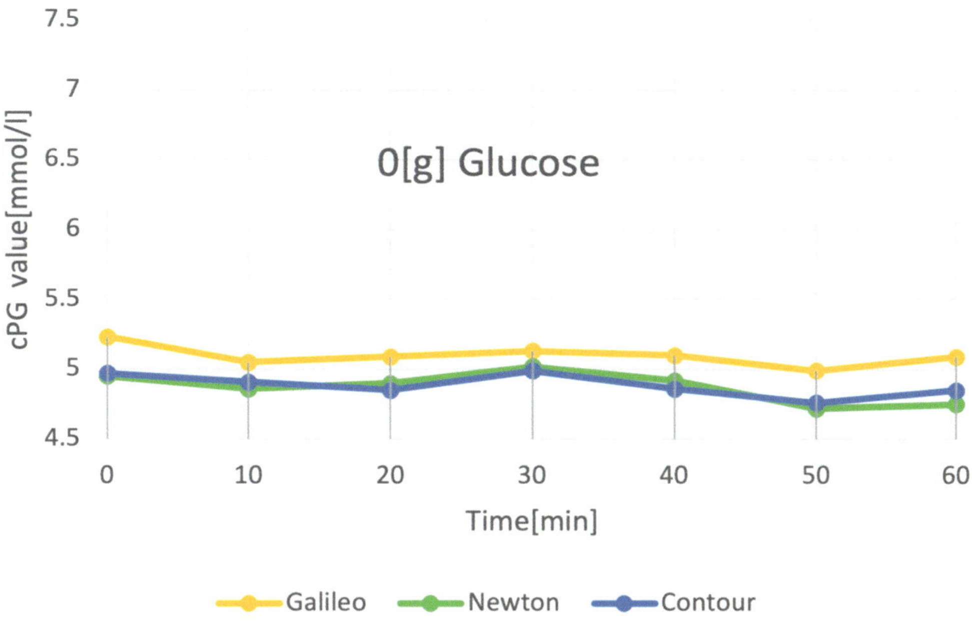

Figure 5.
Mean cPG values for the three GSS systems without any ingested glucose jelly, readings for the control group maintained relatively stable cPG throughout the session The control group maintained relatively stable cPG values, within the normal expected range, between 3.9 and 5.6 mmol/L [14].

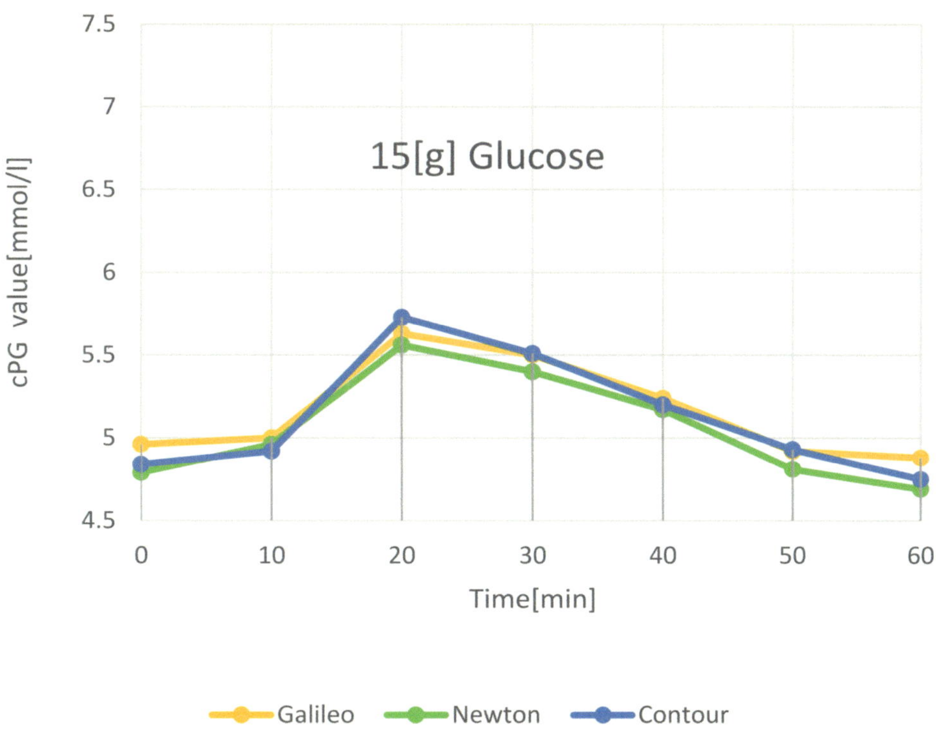

Figure 6.
Mean cPG values for the three GSS systems with 15 g of glucose jelly ingested.

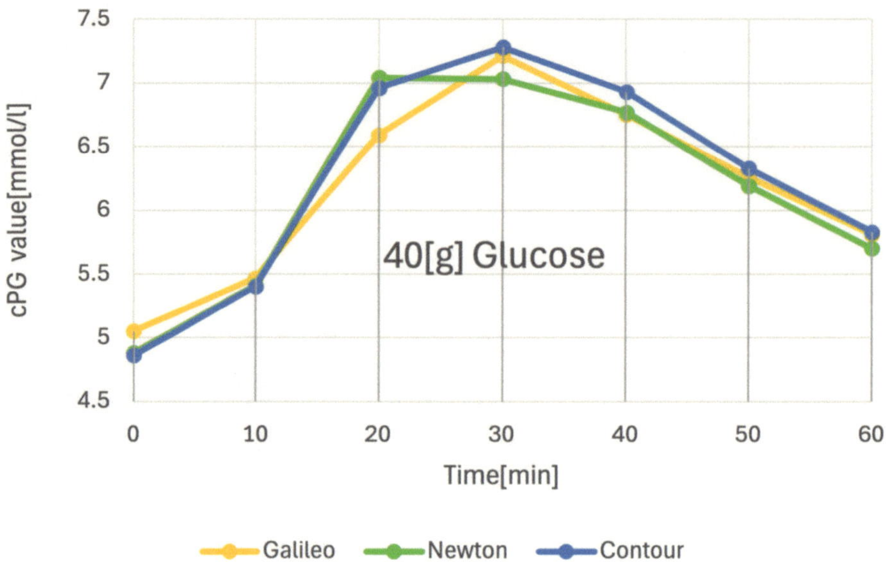

Figure 7.
Mean cPG values for the three GSS systems with 40 g of glucose jelly ingested.

4. Discussion

This chapter is focused on contrasting the accuracy and precision of two GSS, while also looking at the effects of glycemic load and BMI on glycemic response.

4.1 Precision assessment

Both in cases of the control study and the procedures dealing with 15 and 40 g of jelly, the order of precision was found to be consistent: Contour Plus One showed the highest precision, followed by Newton, and finally, Galileo. Following data regarding precision, within the control study (**Table 2**) SD of average triplet value: (1) Contour Plus One (0.079 mmol/L), (2) Newton (0.159 mmol/L), and (3) Galileo (0.169 mmol/L). With respect to the data collected in the study involving the Jelly-shots (**Table 3**) based on the SD of average triplet value: (1) Contour Plus One (0.087 mmol/L), (2) Newton (0.155 mmol/L), and (3) Galileo (0.192 mmol/L). It can hence be inferred that the lowest variability among the results was demonstrated by Contour Plus One. Further, Newton exhibited lower variability in comparison with Galileo.

	Mean	SD	p-value (vs. Contour)
sd Galileo	0.188	0.169	<0.0001
sd Newton	0.251	0.159	<0.0001
sd Contour	0.099	0.079	—

The analysis is based on the data collected from the control study.

Table 2.
Descriptive characteristics of SDs of GSS triplets & P-values.

	Mean	SD	p-value (vs. Contour)
sd Galileo	0.195	0.192	<0.0001
sd Newton	0.254	0.155	<0.0001
sd Contour	0.103	0.087	—

The analysis is based on the data collected from administration of 15 and 40 g glucose-containing jellies.

Table 3.
Descriptive characteristics of SDs of GSS triplets & P-value).

4.2 Accuracy assessment

Using Contour Plus One as the reference device, both Newton and Galileo met the ISO 15197:2013 standards. As shown in **Figures 8** and **9**, the jelly shot studies proved ISO compliance of 98% for Newton and 95% for Galileo. As for the control studies (**Figures 10** and **11**), compliance was 98% for Newton and 97% for Galileo. No statistically significant differences were observed between Newton and Galileo.

4.3 Systemic and random error consideration

Despite the attempts to eliminate systemic errors, it is worth considering that unpredictable random errors may inevitably impact the results. Some of the measures that were taken to minimize systemic errors include:

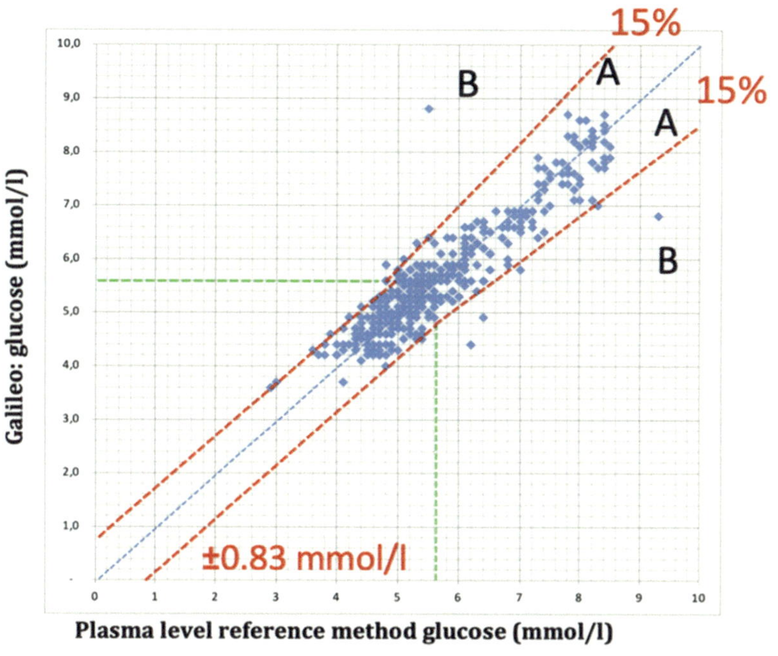

Figure 8.
Consensus Error Grid (CEG) [15] graph plotting Galileo GSS cPG readings against Reference values (Contour Plus One). The readings are from the data collected from the administration of 15 and 40 g glucose-containing jellies. Accuracy shows 402 out of 420 (95%) pairs within the limits of ISO 15197.

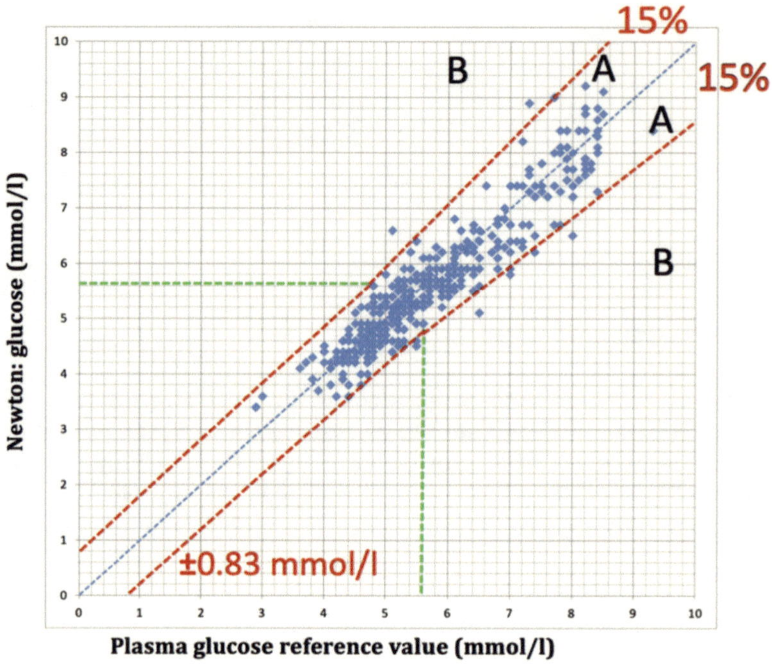

Figure 9.
CEG graph plotting Newton GSS cPG readings against Reference values (Contour Plus One). The readings are from the data collected from the administration of 15 and 40 g glucose-containing jellies. Accuracy shows 412 out of 420 (98%) pairs within the limits of ISO 15197.

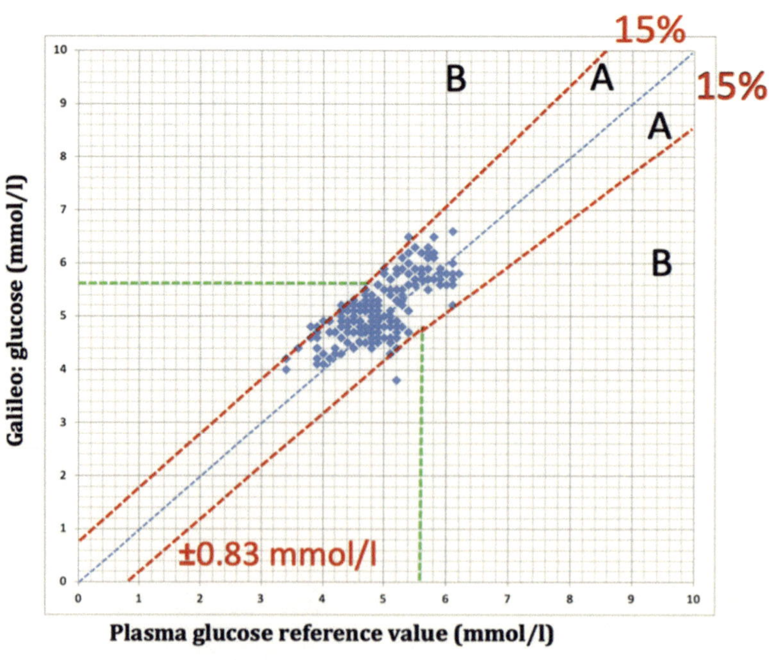

Figure 10.
Consensus Error Grid (CEG) graph plotting Galileo GSS cPG readings against Reference values (Contour Plus One). The readings are from the data collected from the control study. Accuracy shows 204 out of 210 (97%) pairs within limits of ISO 15197.

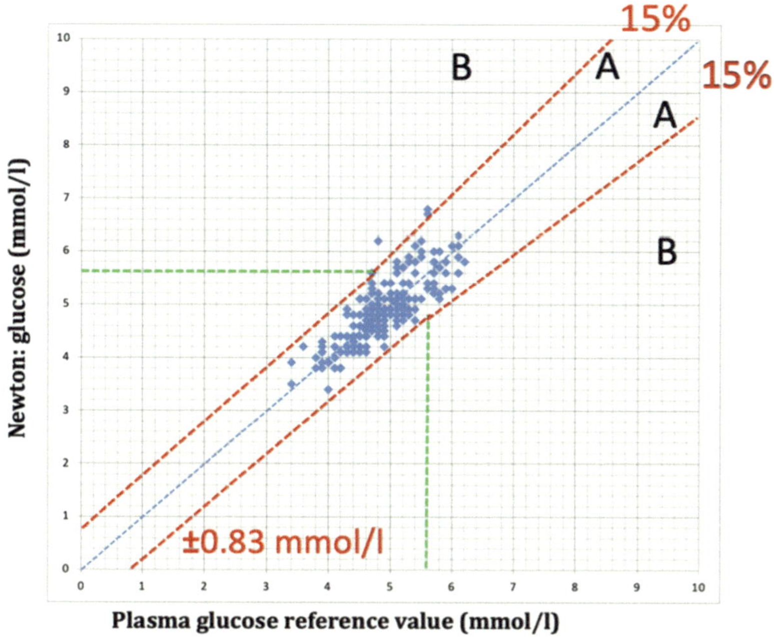

Figure 11.
Consensus Error Grid (CEG) graph plotting Newton GSS cPG readings against Reference values (Contour Plus One). The readings are from the data collected from the control study. Accuracy shows 206 out of 210 (98%) pairs within limits of ISO 15197.

- Participants were thoroughly instructed to wash their hands with soap and water, prior to the finger pricking process.

- During the oral jelly shot administration, volunteers were instructed not to touch, nor have any contact with the jelly container and/or with the administration apparatus, to prevent contamination of the fingers.

- The glucose shots were administered by a single team member, to maintain and ensure consistency [16].

Nevertheless, some systemic errors have occurred that were unaccounted for, which include a single LOT of the Contour Plus One strips being found outdated by 2 months at the time of usage, which raises the question of whether Contour's results were truly the correct choice for reference.

Additionally, some random errors that were difficult to account for include:

- *Environmental conditions*: previous studies have demonstrated deviation and overestimation of cPG by 2.1 mmol/L in case of an increase in temperature by 18°C [17]. This concomitant alteration of reliability should be considered, given that the study was conducted within the morning hours, spanning the time period of November–April (during years 2023/2024), where recorded temperatures range from −8.7 to 8.1°C in Czech Republic, Olomouc region (6–11 am) [18, 19].

- *Strip variability*: Manufacturing differences, specifically in enzyme coating across batches, can impact readings [20].

- *Timing inconsistencies*: delays between lancing and blood application onto the strips can greatly influence the final reading in unpredictable ways due to factors such as blood clotting [21].

- *User technique*: Using a single finger-prick to supply samples for all nine glucometers in each round may have resulted in variability due to insufficient blood volume or contamination with interstitial fluid from squeezing the finger or both, potentially leading to under-reporting of cPG levels [16].

4.4 Strength and weak points of the study

This practice-oriented chapter deals with simple routine testing of various accredited GSS, using a validated GSS (Contour Plus One) as a reference, creating a real-life testing environment (e.g., temperature, user error, and field calibration).

The strength of this study is its independence on other studies to determine reference points while simultaneously building credibility, compliance, and validation of the data. It proves more accessible to patients and clinicians and aids in the reflection of actual patient experience, enhancing the external validity of the study [22].

However, two weak points should be mentioned: (1) throughout the course of the study, the cPG measurements obtained by the GSS were not compared against a laboratory accredited analysis. Instead, a third highly qualified GSS was used as reference. A laboratory accredited analysis refers to measurements performed by a laboratory that has been officially assessed and approved by an official body like the ISO 15197:2013, follows standard procedures, uses calibrated equipment and ensures accuracy [23] and (2) the results and conclusions in this study were based on the assessment of cPG values obtained from participants, where the range of readings fell between 2.9 and 9.3 mmol/L. Further studies, with a wider range of measurements, need to be conducted to support the results that were concluded.

4.5 Glycemic load effect on the glycemic response

As per the data in **Table 1**, which was further plotted in **Figures 5**–7, the time required for the absorptive phase to fully manifest in the circulation and return to baseline can be determined by measuring cPG levels. It can also be determined the maximum increase in cPG for each glycemic load.

To further analyze the cPG values shown in **Table 1**, several observations can be made:

- The mean cPG of the three GSS at the start of the control session (**Figure 5**) was slightly higher (5.05 mmol/l) compared to the other two sessions, 4.86 mmol/L for 15 g and 4.93 mmol/l for 40 g (**Figures 6** and 7). This slight increase is most likely attributed to the Dawn Phenomenon [24], as this session was performed at an earlier time of day.

- Galileo GSS cPG values at the start of the control session (5.23 mmol/L) were significantly higher when compared to the other GSS systems (4.97 and 4.95 mmol/L) (**Figure** 5).

DOI: http://dx.doi.org/10.5772/intechopen.1011456

- The time required to reach maximum cPG after glucose jelly ingestion was influenced by the glucose load; 15 g of glucose jelly caused a peak in cPG values within 20 minutes, whereas 40 g resulted in a peak within 30 minutes (**Figures 6** and 7).
- Newton GSS's maximum cPG value (7.04 mmol/L) for 40 g of glucose was recorded at 20 minutes, which was an exception as the maximum for the other GSS systems (Galileo and Contour Plus One) was recorded at 30 minutes. However, the difference in cPG values at 30 minutes (7.03 mmol/L) and 20 minutes was not significant, with only a slight variation observed between the two time points (0.01 mmol/L).
- Following the ingestion of 15 g of glucose jelly, the cPG values returned to baseline within 50 minutes (**Figure 6**).
- For the 40 g session, cPG values did not return to baseline within the 1-hour period. As supported by source [25], higher glucose loads typically require more time for cPG levels to normalize.

4.6 Correlation between BMI and cPG

As per the results (Section 3.3), Spearman's correlation analysis found a strong negative relationship between cPG increment and BMI when participants did not ingest any glucose jelly after 30 minutes for Galileo (**Table 4**) and after 30 and 50 minutes for Newton (**Tables 5** and **6**). This finding could be related to the procedure in Section 2.1, in which participants were required to fast for a minimum of 8 hours prior to each session. It has been found that an individual's cPG levels when fasting are decreased and will continue to decrease every hour that they continue to fast, thus contributing to lower cPG levels during the participants' fasting session [26]. There was no significant correlation found between cPG increment and BMI using either of the three glucometers when the participants ingested 15 g glucose jelly (**Tables 7–9**). This absence of a significant correlation finding may be related to the

GALILEO, no glucose		Time 10	Time 20	Time 30	Time 40	Time 50	Time 60
BMI (kg/m^2)	Correlation coefficient	−0.579	−0.421	−0.711	−0.281	−0.395	−0.559
	p-value	0.079	0.226	0.021	0.431	0.258	0.093

The measurements span 60 minutes and were measured in 10-minute intervals. Significant findings highlighted.

Table 4.
The correlation between BMI x change in cPG levels without ingesting glucose jelly and using Galileo GSS.

CONTOUR, no glucose		Time 10	Time 20	Time 30	Time 40	Time 50	Time 60
BMI (kg/m^2)	Correlation coefficient	0.293	−0.237	−0.547	0.083	−0.280	−0.444
	p-value	0.412	0.510	0.102	0.821	0.434	0.199

The measurements span 60 minutes and were measured in 10-minute intervals.

Table 5.
The correlation between BMI x change in cPG levels without ingesting glucose jelly and using Contour Plus One.

NEWTON, no glucose		Time 10	Time 20	Time 30	Time 40	Time 50	Time 60
BMI (kg/m^2)	Correlation coefficient	0.082	−0.165	−0.729	−0.485	−0.784	−0.395
	p-value	0.821	0.649	0.017	0.156	0.007	0.58
The measurements span 60 minutes and were measured in 10-minute intervals. Significant findings highlighted.							

Table 6.
The correlation between BMI x change in cPG levels without ingesting glucose jelly and using Newton GSS.

GALILEO, 15 g glucose		Time 10	Time 20	Time 30	Time 40	Time 50	Time 60
BMI (kg/m^2)	Correlation coefficient	0.561	0.333	0.168	−0.061	−0.183	−0.109
	p-value	0.092	0.347	0.642	0.868	0.613	0.763
The measurements span 60 minutes and were measured in 10-minute intervals.							

Table 7.
The correlation between BMI x change in cPG levels ingestion of 15 g glucose jelly and using Galileo GSS.

CONTOUR, 15 g glucose		Time 10	Time 20	Time 30	Time 40	Time 50	Time 60
BMI (kg/m^2)	Correlation coefficient	0.131	0.190	−0.043	−0.231	0.140	−0.061
	p-value	0.717	0.600	0.907	0.521	0.699	0.868
The measurements span 60 minutes and were measured in 10-minute intervals.							

Table 8.
The correlation between BMI x change in cPG levels ingestion of 15 g glucose jelly and using Contour Plus One.

NEWTON, 15 g glucose		Time 10	Time 20	Time 30	Time 40	Time 50	Time 60
BMI (kg/m^2)	Correlation coefficient	0.237	0.359	0.328	−0.140	0.529	0.438
	p-value	0.510	0.309	0.354	0.700	0.116	0.206
The measurements span 60 minutes and were measured in 10-minute intervals.							

Table 9.
The correlation between BMI x change in cPG levels ingestion of 15 g glucose jelly and using Newton GSS.

smaller GL of 15 g glucose jelly. There have been findings that concluded that lower GL foods are not as effective at raising cPG levels as higher GL foods [11].

Finally, Spearman's correlation analysis found a strong positive correlation between cPG increment and BMI when participants ingested 40 g glucose jelly after 40 and 50 minutes for the Newton GSS and after 50 minutes for the Galileo GSS (**Tables 10–12**). As shown in the graphs (**Figures 12–14**), participants with a BMI of at least 25 had poorer glycemic responses when 40 g glucose jelly was ingested, as opposed to participants with lower BMI values. These findings may contribute to the thought that individuals with a higher BMI have a less adequate response to glucose than those with a lower BMI, or that having a higher BMI may influence the glucose jelly absorption rates, which in turn influence the cPG levels. There have also been

NEWTON, 40 g glucose		Time 10	Time 20	Time 30	Time 40	Time 50	Time 60
BMI (kg/m^2)	Correlation coefficient	−0.334	−0.012	−0.088	0.486	0.663	0.529
	p-value	0.345	0.973	0.808	0.154	0.037	0.116

The measurements span 60 minutes and were measured in 10-minute intervals. Significant findings highlighted.

Table 10.
The correlation between BMI x change in cPG levels ingestion of 40 g glucose jelly and using Galileo GSS.

CONTOUR, 40 g glucose		Time 10	Time 20	Time 30	Time 40	Time 50	Time 60
BMI (kg/m^2)	Correlation coefficient	−0.036	−0.143	0.055	0.547	0.523	0.511
	p-value	0.920	0.693	0.881	0.102	0.121	0.132

The measurements span 60 minutes and were measured in 10-minute intervals.

Table 11.
The correlation between BMI x change in cPG levels ingestion of 40 g glucose jelly and using Contour Plus One.

NEWTON, 40 g glucose		Time 10	Time 20	Time 30	Time 40	Time 50	Time 60
BMI (kg/m^2)	Correlation coefficient	−0.018	−0.085	-0.079	0.687	0.668	0.389
	p-value	0.960	0.815	0.828	0.028	0.035	0.266

The measurements span 60 minutes and were measured in 10-minute intervals. Significant findings highlighted.

Table 12.
The correlation between BMI x change in cPG levels ingestion of 40 g glucose jelly and using Newton GSS.

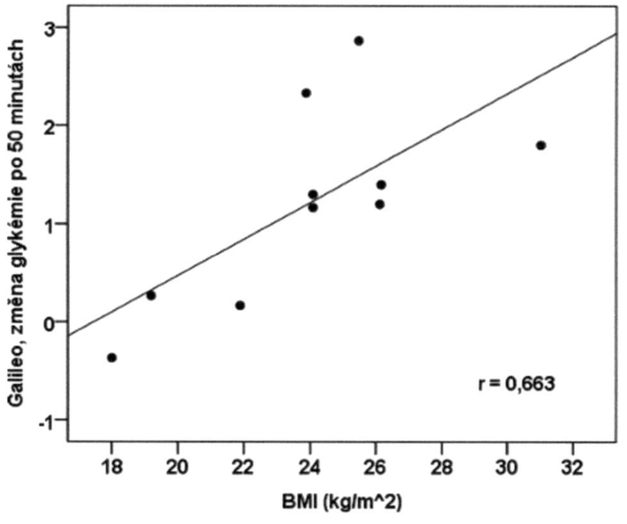

Figure 12.
Correlation between cPG increment x BMI after 50 minutes using Galileo GSS.

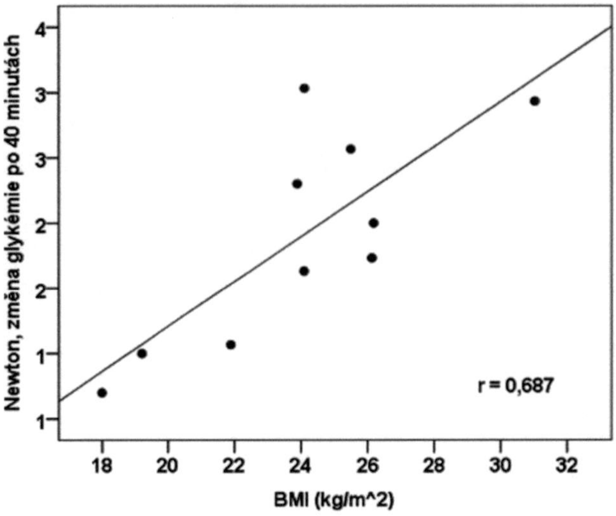

Figure 13.
Correlation between cPG increment x BMI after 40 minutes using Newton GSS.

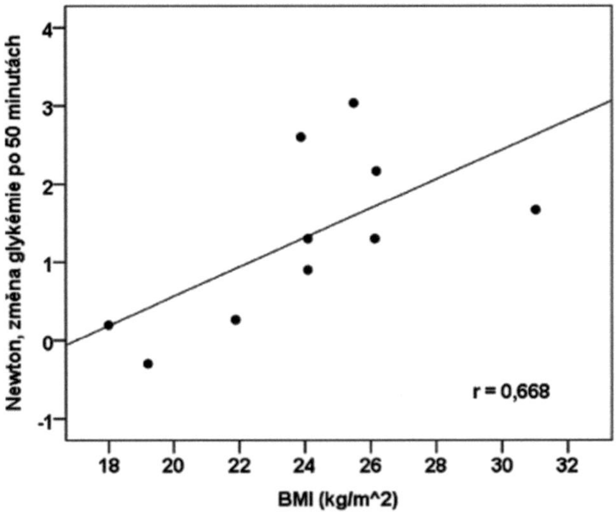

Figure 14.
Correlation between cPG increment x BMI after 50 minutes using Newton GSS.

links between obesity and insulin resistance, which affects glycemic response negatively; this supports the finding that those with a higher BMI also had a diminished glucose response [27].

Although it is true that certain factors could not be fully controlled or accounted for, the study represents a valuable step toward a better and deeper understanding of different glucometer devices. The study strives to highlight and address key areas and aspects open for investigation and improvement within this important field. Furthermore, the negative relationship between cPG increment and BMI in fasting patients who did not ingest glucose, may suggest that there are more significant factors to consider when looking at an individual's response to glucose. Lastly, through looking at the effects of glycemic load on individuals, it is of most importance to note that during a state of hypoglycemia, the consumption of an adequate amount of glucose can be lifesaving [28].

5. Summary and conclusion

Firstly, with regards to accuracy, there was no significant difference between Gallio and Newton, and they both met ISO 15197:2013 criteria. As for precision, Contour had the least variability among its readings, followed by Newton and then Galileo. When considering the effects of GL on glycemic response, it was determined that a larger GL contributes to a greater elevation of cPG levels. Finally, when looking at the correlation between BMI and glycemic response, it was found that a higher BMI contributes to a greater elevation of cPG levels as well. Although the results of the study were as predicted and rather positive, any future relative studies should have a larger participant group with a wider range of BMI levels, as having more varied data would be beneficial and aid in further cementing the above conclusions.

Acknowledgements

Authors' contributions: B.M. was in charge of the manuscript and procedural design, in addition to measuring cPG from a single finger-prick. J.A. was responsible for recording progress in the form of images and videos, administration of the glucose-containing jelly, and reviewing the text. Ab.A. was responsible for cPG data collection. A.A. was responsible for reloading the strips in the glucometers. S.S. was responsible for the measurement of the height and weight of volunteers as well as preparation of them for the procedures. O.M. was responsible for keeping track of the time and workflow of the procedures. This chapter is a result of collective and cooperative efforts. Our gratitude goes toward the volunteers who participated in this study.

Our deepest gratitude goes to MUDr. Martin Nezval, Dr. Mgr. Jana Zaplatalová, the Department of Internal Medicine II – Gastroenterology and Geriatrics, University Hospital Olomouc, the Department of Physiology, along with the Department of Biophysics, Faculty of Medicine and Dentistry, Palacký University Olomouc, Czech Republic.

Abbreviations

BMI	body mass index
CEG	Consensus Error Grid
cPG	capillary plasma glucose
GDH-FAD	glucose dehydrogenase-flavin adenine dinucleotide
GI	glycemic index
GL	glycemic load
GSS	glucometer-strips systems
SD	standard deviation

Author details

Biayni Minasyan*, Jenna Al-Hammady, Abdullah Ahmed, Alexia Assaad, Serdar Serdar and Olufunmilayo Moronwiyan
Department of Physiology, Faculty of Medicine and Dentistry, Palacky University Olomouc, Czech Republic

*Address all correspondence to: biayni.minasyan@gmail.com

References

[1] The Diabetes Control and Complications Trial Research Group. The effect of intensive treatment of diabetes on the development and progression of long-term complications in insulin-dependent diabetes mellitus. New England Journal of Medicine. 1993;**329**(14):977-986. DOI: 10.1056/NEJM199309303291401

[2] D'Orazio P et al. Approved IFCC recommendation on reporting results for blood glucose. Clinical Chemistry. 2005;**51**(9):15731576. DOI: 10.1373/clinchem.2005.051672

[3] International Organization for Standardization. ISO 15197:2013 - In Vitro Diagnostic Test Systems — Requirements for Blood-Glucose Monitoring Systems for Self-Testing in Managing Diabetes Mellitus. 2013. Available from: https://www.iso.org/standard/54976.html

[4] Today's Clinical Lab. How Accurate Is POC Glucose Testing? 2022. Available from: https://www.clinicallab.com/how-accurate-is-poc-glucose-testing-169

[5] Tang Z, Louie RF, Lee JH, Lee DM, Miller EE, Kost GJ. Oxygen effects on glucose meter measurements with glucosedehydrogenase-and oxidase-based test strips for point-of-care testing. Critical Care Medicine. 2001;**29**(5):1062-1070. DOI: 10.1097/00003246-200105000-00038

[6] Weissenbacher S, Yang C-Y, Kuan T-C, Demircik F, Hanna M, Pfützner A. System accuracy assessments with a blood glucose meter with combined glucose and ß-hydroxybutyrate measurement capabilities. Expert Review of Molecular Diagnostics. 2019;**19**(11):1043-1048. DOI: 10.1080/14737159.2019.1662300

[7] International Organization for Standardization (ISO). ISO 15197:2013(E): In Vitro Diagnostic Test Systems—Requirements for Blood-Glucose Monitoring Systems for Self-Testing in Managing Diabetes Mellitus. Geneva, Switzerland: International Organization for Standardization; 2013. Available from: https://www.iso.org/standard/54976.html [last reviewed and confirmed 2018]

[8] Caswell M, Brown D, Frank J, Wallace JF, Pardo S. Accuracy and user performance evaluation of a blood glucose monitoring system which wirelessly transmits results to compatible insulin pumps: Evaluation of the CONTOUR PLUS LINK 2.4 blood glucose monitoring system, assessed according to ISO 15197:2013 criteria. Current Medical Research and Opinion. 2020;**36**(5):757-764. DOI: 10.1080/03007995.2020.1734919

[9] Klaff L, Shelat P, Zondorak D, Wayland-Smith A, Vernes P, Richardson JM. Accuracy and user performance of a new blood glucose monitoring system. Journal of Diabetes Science and Technology. 2021;**15**(6):1382-1389. DOI: 10.1177/1932296820974348. Epub 2020 Nov 26

[10] Galgani J, Aguirre C, Díaz E. Acute effect of meal glycemic index and glycemic load on blood glucose and insulin responses in humans. Nutrition Journal. 2006;**5**:22. DOI: 10.1186/1475-2891-5-22

[11] Yalçın T, Al A, Rakıcıoğlu N. The effects of meal glycemic load on blood glucose levels of adults with different

body mass indexes. Indian Journal of Endocrinology and Metabolism. 2017;**21**(1):71-75. DOI: 10.4103/2230-8210.195995

[12] Wellion. Wellion 1Shot. Austria, Burgenland: Wellion; 1997. Available from: https://www.wellion.eu/en/products/invert-sugar-syrup/wellion-1shot [Accessed: April 12, 2025]

[13] Wellion. Wellion Gold. Austria, Burgenland: Wellion; 1997. Available from: https://www.wellion.eu/en/products/wellionvet/wellion-gold [Accessed: April 12, 2025]

[14] World Health Organization. Mean Fasting Blood Glucose. 2025. Available from: https://www.who.int/data/gho/indicator-metadata-registry/imr-details/2380# [Accessed: April 17, 2025]

[15] Tian T, Aaron RE, Kohn MA, Klonoff DC. The need for a modern error grid for clinical accuracy of blood glucose monitors and continuous glucose monitors. Journal of Diabetes Science and Technology. 2024;**18**(1):3-9. DOI: 10.1177/19322968231214281

[16] Lacher DA et al. Effects of improper testing techniques on the accuracy of glucose meters. Clinical Chemistry and Laboratory Medicine. 2011;**49**(12):1931-1936. DOI: 10.1515/CCLM.2011.874

[17] Miao Y et al. Adverse impact of temperature and humidity on blood glucose monitoring reliability: A pilot study. Diabetes Technology & Therapeutics. 2007;**9**(1):1-9. DOI: 10.1089/dia.2006.0051

[18] Accu-Chek. Factors Affecting Accuracy and the Importance of Interference Testing. UK & Ireland; n.d. Available from: https://www.accu-chek.co.uk/hcp/resources/factors-affecting-accuracy: Accu-Chek [Accessed: April 14, 2025]

[19] Time and Date. Past Weather in Olomouc, Czechia — November 2023 to April 2024. Norway, Stavanger: Time and Date; n.d. Available from: https://www.timeanddate.com/weather/czech-republic/olomouc/historic [Accessed: April 14, 2025]

[20] Rebrin K et al. Accuracy and consistency of blood glucose test strips in multiple batches. Journal of Diabetes Science and Technology. 2005;**1**(3):281-285

[21] Mahmoodpoor A, Hamishehkar H, Shadvar K, Sanaie S, Iranpour A, Fattahi V. Validity of bedside blood glucose measurement in critically ill patients with intensive insulin therapy. Indian Journal of Critical Care Medicine. 2016;**20**(11):653-657. DOI: 10.4103/0972-5229.194009

[22] King F, Ahn D, Hsiao V, Porco T, Klonoff DC. A review of blood glucose monitor accuracy. Diabetes Technology & Therapeutics. 2018;**20**:843-856. DOI: 10.1089/dia.2018.0232

[23] Hunt BE et al. Validity and reliability of a glucometer against industry reference standards. Journal of Diabetes Science and Technology. 2014;**8**(1):95-99. Available from: https://journals.sagepub.com/doi/abs/10.1177/1932296813514315

[24] Porcellati F, Lucidi P, Bolli GB, Fanelli CG. Thirty years of research on the dawn phenomenon: Lessons to optimize blood glucose control in diabetes. Diabetes Care. 2013;**36**(12):3860-3862. DOI: 10.2337/dc13-2088

[25] Cassady BA, McDonald JD, Yalawar M, Baggs GE, Maki KC. Pilot study on the impact of a carbohydrate

loading drink on postprandial glycemic responses and gastric emptying in adults with prediabetes and type 2 diabetes mellitus. Nutrition in Clinical Practice. 2023;**38**:108-117. DOI: 10.1002/ncp.10845

[26] Moebus S, Göres L, Lösch C, Jöckel K-H. Impact of time since last caloric intake on blood glucose levels. European Journal of Epidemeology. 2011;**26**(9):719-728. DOI: 10.1007/s10654-011-9609-z

[27] Kahn BB, Flier JS. Obesity and insulin resistance. Journal of Clinical Investigation. 2000;**106**(4):473-481. DOI: 10.1172/jci10842

[28] Villani M, de Courten B, Zoungas S. Emergency treatment of hypoglycaemia: A guideline and evidence review. Diabetic Medicine. 2017;**34**(9):1205-1211. DOI: 10.1111/dme.13379. Epub 2017 Jun 29

Section 2

Management of Type 2 Diabetes and Its Complications

Chapter 3

Exercise and Type 2 Diabetes Mellitus

Ahmed Ahmed and Samah Ismail

Abstract

Exercise is a crucial component of lifestyle therapy for both the prevention and management of type 2 diabetes (T2D). The aim of this chapter is to explain the various exercises implemented for the management of diabetic patients. These recommendations stem from strong evidence linking physical activity to a reduced risk of developing T2D, improved disease management, and lower diabetes-related morbidity and mortality. However, individuals with T2D face physiological and behavioral challenges that can hinder their ability to fully reap the benefits of physical activity. Physiological barriers include diabetes-related impairments in exercise capacity, higher perceived exertion at lower workloads, and the need for careful glycemic management during physical activity. Additionally, social and psychological factors, such as depression and low self-efficacy, can further discourage participation in exercise. Individual responses to physical activity can vary based on factors like sex, genetics, and environmental influences, making it difficult to predict the specific benefits for each person. The optimal exercise dosage, duration, timing, and type for maximizing health outcomes remain unclear. Both aerobic and resistance training enhance insulin action, at least in the short term, and can aid in managing blood glucose levels, lipids, blood pressure, cardiovascular risk, mortality, and overall quality of life. However, to sustain these benefits, exercise must be performed consistently and should ideally incorporate a variety of training types.

Keywords: exercise, training, aerobic, resistance, HIIT

1. Introduction

Diabetes mellitus causes both macrovascular and microvascular complications, which can lead to severe health issues. Regular exercise is a key component of diabetes management, offering significant therapeutic benefits. In individuals with diabetes, exercise supports cardiovascular health by lowering the risk of heart disease and mortality, aids in weight management, and enhances glycemic control. Improved tissue sensitivity to insulin further contributes to better plasma glucose concentration regulation [1]. The purpose of this chapter is to explain the various exercises implemented for the management of diabetic patients.

1.1 Types of exercise and physical activity

Aerobic exercise involves continuous, repetitive movements of large muscle groups, such as walking, cycling, jogging, and swimming, which primarily utilize aerobic energy systems. Resistance training, or strength training, includes activities using free weights, weight machines, body mass, or resistance bands to build muscle strength. Flexibility exercises enhance joint range of motion, while balance exercises improve gait stability and help prevent falls. Activities such as tai chi and yoga integrate flexibility, balance, and resistance training [2].

1.2 Aerobic exercise benefits

Engaging in aerobic exercise enhances mitochondrial density, insulin sensitivity, oxidative enzyme activity, vascular function, lung capacity, immune response, and cardiac output [3]. A moderate to high volume of aerobic activity significantly reduces cardiovascular and overall mortality risks in both type 1 and type 2 diabetes [4]. For individuals with type 2 diabetes, it helps lower A1C, blood pressure, and insulin resistance [5]. High-intensity interval training (HIIT) is particularly effective for quickly enhancing muscle oxidative capacity, insulin sensitivity, and glycemic control in type 2 diabetes [6].

1.3 Resistance exercise benefits

Diabetes is linked to reduced muscle strength and a faster decline in physical function [7, 8]. Resistance training benefits all adults by increasing muscle mass, body composition, strength, functional capacity, mental well-being, bone density, insulin sensitivity, blood pressure regulation, lipid profiles, and cardiovascular health [3]. In type 2 diabetes, resistance training supports glycemic control, improves insulin resistance, reduces fat mass and blood pressure, and enhances strength and lean muscle mass [9].

1.4 Other physical activity benefits

Flexibility and balance exercises are especially important for older adults with diabetes, as joint mobility may decline due to aging and hyperglycemia-related effects [10]. Stretching increases flexibility and joint range of motion [11] but does not directly impact glycemic control. Balance training, however, can lower the risk of falls, even for individuals with peripheral neuropathy [12]. Group exercises incorporating resistance and balance training, as well as tai chi, have been shown to decrease fall rates [13]. Yoga and tai chi may improve glycemic control, lipid profiles, body composition, and overall quality of life in people with diabetes, though further research is needed [14].

2. Exercise for glycemic control

Research on the effects of exercise on glycemic control has largely focused on aerobic exercise for individuals with prediabetes or type 2 diabetes (T2D). Aerobic activities, which include walking, jogging, running, and cycling, involve rhythmic movements of large muscle groups. This form of exercise improves insulin sensitivity, vascular function, aerobic fitness, and body fat reduction [2]. Guidelines from the American College of Sports Medicine (ACSM) and the American Diabetes Association (ADA) suggest engaging in at least 150 minutes per week of moderate-to-vigorous aerobic exercise, spread over at least 3 days, with no more than two consecutive days without activity. The rationale for this frequency is that aerobic exercise enhances insulin sensitivity, an effect that persists for up to 48 hours post-exercise [15, 16].

Skeletal muscle plays a crucial role in glycemic regulation, facilitating blood glucose uptake through both insulin-dependent and -independent pathways. During aerobic exercise, glucose transporter type 4 (GLUT-4) moves to the cell membrane, increasing glucose uptake without insulin [17]. This effect diminishes within 3–6 hours, after which muscles exhibit heightened insulin sensitivity, lasting up to 48 hours depending on factors, such as intensity, diet, and sleep [18]. Notably, aerobic exercise lowers the risk of hypoglycemia in T2D patients who do not use insulin and contributes to overall cardiovascular health, irrespective of weight loss [4].

Substantial evidence supports the role of exercise in improving glycemic control. A six-month aerobic training study involving overweight individuals with T2D, consisting of four sessions per week (45–60 minutes per session at 50–75% of peak oxygen uptake (VO2peak)), resulted in decreased fasting plasma glucose (−1.03 mmol/l) and insulin levels (−20.2 pmol/l) compared to a non-exercising control group [19]. Similarly, a 12–16-week aerobic exercise program (60 minutes at ~75% VO2peak, 4–5 days per week) led to a reduction in fasting blood glucose (−0.35 mmol/l) and increased insulin sensitivity in individuals with impaired glucose tolerance or T2D [20]. These improvements are significant since a 1% decrease in glycated hemoglobin (HbA1c) is associated with a 21% reduction in diabetes-related mortality [21]. Furthermore, a meta-analysis of 12 aerobic and two resistance training trials found a 10 mmol/mol decrease in post-intervention HbA1c in exercise groups compared to controls, independent of weight loss [22].

Recent advancements, such as continuous glucose monitoring (CGM), provide better insights into acute glycemic changes. A meta-analysis of 11 aerobic and resistance exercise interventions demonstrated that exercise significantly lowered average glucose concentrations (−0.8 mmol/l) and reduced the time spent in hyperglycemic ranges by approximately 129 minutes daily [23]. Aerobic exercise also offers cardiovascular benefits, as shown in a meta-analysis of 1003 T2D patients, which found reductions in systolic (−5.6 mmHg) and diastolic (−5.5 mmHg) blood pressure (−0.3 mmol/l), and total cholesterol (−0.3 mmol/l) [5].

While aerobic and resistance exercises have unique health benefits, incorporating both forms of training may enhance adherence and optimize outcomes. Given that T2D is associated with reduced muscle strength and accelerated muscle loss, resistance training is valuable for maintaining muscle mass and functional status [9]. Resistance training involves muscle contractions against external forces using weights, machines, body mass, or resistance bands. ACSM and ADA guidelines recommend resistance training at least 2–3 nonconsecutive days per week, with intensity levels determined by the number of repetitions performed per set (reps per set). Moderate training typically involves 10–15 reps per set, while vigorous training comprises 6–8 reps per set [2].

Resistance training significantly benefits glycemic control, muscle strength, bone density, and muscle quality. A meta-analysis of over 8500 T2D patients found a − 9.26 mmol/mol reduction in HbA1c following structured resistance training. While this reduction is clinically meaningful, resistance training primarily affects postprandial rather than fasting glucose levels [24]. Skeletal muscle accounts for ~80% of insulin-mediated glucose uptake [25], making resistance exercise a strategic approach for blood glucose regulation. A separate meta-analysis of 14 studies confirmed that resistance training lowers total cholesterol, low-density lipoprotein (LDL) cholesterol, and triacylglycerols [26]. Additionally, a six-month high-intensity resistance training program for older T2D patients reduced both systolic and diastolic blood pressure [27].

Combining aerobic and resistance training appears to offer the most comprehensive benefits. A combined regimen of 30 minutes of aerobic exercise (40–80% heart rate reserve) plus 30 minutes of resistance training (40–60% of one-rep max) resulted in significant reductions in fasting blood glucose (−2 mmol/l) and triacylglycerols (−5.9 mmol/l), along with increases in fat-free mass (+0.4 kg) [28]. A meta-analysis of 915 participants across 14 trials found that concurrent training produced greater reductions in HbA1c (−2.67 mmol/mol), fasting glucose (−1.94 mmol/l), and triacylglycerols (−0.28 mmol/l) than aerobic or resistance training alone [29]. Trials, such as the Health Benefits of Aerobic and Resistance Training in Individuals with Type 2 Diabetes (HART-D) and the Diabetes Aerobic and Resistance Exercise (DARE) study, further confirm the effectiveness of concurrent training in reducing HbA1c and improving cardiovascular health [30].

The HART-D trial was specifically designed to ensure that exercise volume was comparable across different workout modalities. The study included aerobic training (12 kcal/kg/week or 50 kJ/week at 50–80% VO2max), resistance training (three sessions per week consisting of two sets of four upper-body exercises, three sets of three leg exercises, and two sets of abdominal crunches and back extensions), and a combined regimen (10 kcal/kg/week or 42 kJ/week of aerobic exercise plus two sessions of one set of the resistance exercises mentioned). The results showed that only the combined training approach significantly reduced HbA1c levels compared to the control group, with a decrease of 0.34% [31].

This finding aligns with the Italian Diabetes and Exercise Study (IDES), which demonstrated that combining aerobic and resistance exercises is effective in lowering HbA1c, LDL cholesterol, and blood pressure compared to standard care [32]. It also supports evidence that short-term, high-intensity functional training, such as CrossFit, can enhance insulin sensitivity and pancreatic function in individuals with type 2 diabetes (T2D) [33]. While the exact mechanisms behind exercise-induced improvements in pancreatic function, potential factors include increased GLUT-2 (glucose transporter type 2) transporter content, enhanced protein kinase B (Akt) signaling, and greater glucokinase activity. Additionally, mitochondrial function in beta cells may play a role, and muscle-released cytokines could influence beta-cell mass or function [34, 35]. Overall, these studies reinforce the current recommendations from the American College of Sports Medicine (ACSM) and the American Diabetes Association (ADA), which advocate for concurrent training and at least 2 days of resistance training per week as part of a minimum of 150 minutes of moderate-intensity exercise to effectively regulate plasma glucose levels [36].

2.1 High-intensity interval training (HIIT) and glycemic control

Despite the well-established benefits of exercise for glycemic control, many individuals cite time constraints as a barrier to consistent physical activity [37]. HIIT has emerged as a time-efficient alternative that enhances glycemic control and cardiovascular health. HIIT involves short bursts of high-intensity exercise (e.g., 75–95% HRmax) interspersed with recovery periods (30–60% HRmax). Unlike continuous training, HIIT allows individuals to achieve substantial health benefits in less time [38]. However, it may not be suitable for all individuals due to its intensity, and caution should be exercised to minimize the risk of injury or exercise-induced hypoglycemia, particularly among insulin users [39]. Therefore, individuals who are medically approved for vigorous exercise may benefit from HIIT as an alternative to traditional moderate-intensity workouts [40].

Interval training involves alternating between exercise and recovery phases. In HIIT, individuals perform high-intensity aerobic exercise (ranging from 10 seconds to 4 minutes at 75–95% HRmax) interspersed with active or passive recovery periods (lasting 12 seconds to 5 minutes at 30–60% HRmax). Unlike traditional continuous exercise, where intensity remains steady, HIIT elicits heart rate responses of approximately 75–95% HRmax. Current ACSM guidelines recommend at least 75 minutes of vigorous activity per week, with no more than two consecutive days between sessions [2].

Research indicates that HIIT, similar to continuous high-intensity exercise, supports glycemic control [36]. Short-term HIIT studies, including six sessions of 10 × 60-second cycling bouts at ~90% HRmax over 2 weeks, have demonstrated reductions in 24-hour blood glucose levels measured by CGM [41]. Additionally, muscle biopsies revealed improved mitochondrial capacity, indicating enhanced oxidative glucose utilization.

Pancreatic function improvements have also been observed following an 8-week HIIT cycling intervention in individuals with T2D (three weekly sessions of 10 × 60-second cycling at ~90% HRmax). Compared to a healthy control group, participants showed reductions in fasting glucose, HbA1c, HOMA-IR (Homeostatic Model Assessment of Insulin Resistance) (a measure of insulin resistance), HOMA-b (Homeostatic Model Assessment of Beta-Cell Function) (an index of insulin secretion), and abdominal fat mass [42].

A meta-analysis of ~1400 individuals with T2D found that HIIT yielded greater improvements in HbA1c, HOMA-IR, fasting serum glucose, and VO2peak compared to moderate- and low-intensity exercise [43]. However, differences in total energy expenditure among groups were not standardized, possibly influencing exercise adaptations across intensities. Nevertheless, an 8-week HIIT program (three weekly cycling sessions at 80–110% of peak power output) increased aerobic capacity while reducing blood insulin concentrations and HOMA-IR in adults with T2D, relative to non-insulin-resistant, non-obese controls [44]. Collectively, these findings suggest that HIIT is an effective strategy for improving glycemic control in individuals with T2D [36].

The question of whether HIIT is superior to continuous training remains unresolved. In a study comparing 11 weeks of HIIT (10 one-minute intervals at 95% peak workload with one-minute active recovery) to continuous endurance training (40 minutes of cycling at 50% peak workload, 3 days per week), HIIT led to greater improvements in VO2max while yielding similar effects on HbA1c, fasting glucose, postprandial glucose, and HOMA-IR in individuals with T2D—despite requiring less time and energy expenditure [45].

These findings align with a recent meta-analysis of 13 HIIT trials involving 345 patients with T2D, which found significant reductions in HbA1c (−6 mmol/mol mean difference) compared to a non-exercise control group. However, there were no significant differences between HIIT and continuous training in terms of HOMA-IR or cardiovascular disease (CVD) risk reduction [46].

Additionally, a 12-week HIIT cycling program (one four-minute bout at 90% VO2peak, three sessions per week) reduced pulse wave velocity (PWV), a measure of arterial stiffness, and improved systolic blood pressure to levels comparable to those achieved with moderate-intensity continuous training (MICT) [47]. Flow-mediated dilation (FMD), an indicator of endothelial function, also showed similar improvements between HIIT and MICT [48].

While aerobic HIIT has primarily been studied using treadmill or cycling exercises, recent research has begun exploring resistance-based HIIT for improving fitness and glycemic control. In a year-long study, individuals performing resistance HIIT (10–12 repetitions of upper- and lower-body exercises at 90% heart rate reserve [HRR], followed by one-minute rest at 40–60% HRR, three times per week) showed greater vascular benefits than those performing moderate-intensity resistance training. Both groups experienced reductions in carotid intima-media thickness (cIMT), an indicator of carotid atherosclerosis, but only HIIT led to a decrease in PWV, suggesting reduced arterial stiffness [49]. Further studies are needed to determine the optimal combination of resistance and aerobic HIIT for maximizing glycemic control in individuals with T2D [36].

3. Effects of physical activity on insulin action

Both acute and long-term exercise training influence insulin action in muscle and liver [50]. Aerobic exercise significantly increases muscle glucose uptake, initially through insulin-independent mechanisms, with post-exercise effects lasting up to 48 hours via both insulin-dependent and -independent pathways [51–53]. Shorter, more intense exercise sessions can also enhance insulin action for 24 hours, while low-intensity exercise for at least 60 minutes benefits insulin-resistant individuals [54, 55]. Aerobic exercise, even at low intensity for at least 60 minutes, can improve insulin sensitivity in obese, insulin-resistant adults for up to 24 hours [56]. If the primary objective is to enhance insulin action, engaging in daily moderate- or high-intensity exercise is likely the most effective approach [18]. Both aerobic and resistance training induce beneficial adaptations in skeletal muscle, adipose tissue, and the liver, improving insulin sensitivity even in the absence of weight loss [57, 58]. Regular aerobic exercise enhances muscle insulin sensitivity in individuals with type 2 diabetes, with improvements correlating to exercise volume [59]. Even low-volume exercise, burning as little as 400 kcal or 1673 kJ per week, can enhance insulin action in previously sedentary adults, with the greatest benefits seen in those with higher baseline insulin resistance [60]. A dose-response relationship exists up to approximately 2500 kcal or 10,460 kJ per week [60].

Resistance training similarly improves insulin sensitivity [57], as do HIIT and other exercise modalities [5, 41, 61]. Combining endurance and resistance training may yield even greater benefits [30], and HIIT may offer advantages over continuous aerobic exercise in individuals with diabetes [6].

3.1 Physical activity for adults with type 2 diabetes

The Look AHEAD trial examined the effects of an intensive lifestyle intervention, including at least 175 minutes of weekly exercise, compared to standard diabetes care [62]. As reviewed by Pi-Sunyer [63], the intensive lifestyle intervention group demonstrated significantly greater and sustained improvements in weight loss, cardiorespiratory fitness, blood glucose regulation, blood pressure, and lipid levels while requiring fewer medications. Additionally, they experienced lower rates of sleep apnea, severe diabetic kidney disease, retinopathy, depression, sexual dysfunction, urinary incontinence, and knee pain. They also maintained better physical mobility and quality of life, all while reducing overall healthcare costs. This trial provided compelling evidence of the substantial health benefits associated with intensive lifestyle intervention.

Furthermore, aerobic exercise is particularly effective in improving glycemic control in individuals with type 2 diabetes, especially when performed for at least 150 minutes per week [24]. Resistance training, whether using free weights or weight machines, enhances strength in adults with type 2 diabetes by approximately 50% [23] and reduces A1C levels by 9.2 mmol/mol [9, 24]. A meta-analysis of 12 studies found that aerobic exercise led to a slightly greater reduction in A1C (by −2.9 mmol/mol) compared to resistance training, although both forms of exercise had similar effects on cardiovascular risk markers [64]. Notably, a combination of aerobic and resistance training is more effective for glycemic control than either type alone [31]. Therefore, for optimal glycemic management and overall health benefits, adults with type 2 diabetes should ideally engage in both aerobic and resistance exercises [2].

3.2 Recommended physical activity for individuals with diabetes

3.2.1 General recommendations

- Medical clearance is generally not required for asymptomatic individuals before starting low- to moderate-intensity activities, such as brisk walking.

- Most adults with diabetes should engage in at least 150 minutes per week of moderate-to-vigorous intensity exercise, spread over at least 3 days, with no more than two consecutive days without exercise. Shorter durations (75 minutes per week) of vigorous-intensity training may suffice for younger, physically fit individuals.

- Children and adolescents with diabetes should aim for at least 60 minutes of moderate-to-vigorous aerobic activity daily, incorporating muscle-strengthening and bone-strengthening exercises at least three times per week.

- Adults should participate in resistance training at least two to three times per week on nonconsecutive days.

- Older adults should include flexibility and balance training two to three times per week, with activities like yoga and tai chi as options.

- Increasing overall daily movement, even through non-exercise activities, is encouraged.

- Supervised exercise programs offer greater health benefits compared to unsupervised training.

3.3 Pre-exercise screening and health considerations

The American College of Sports Medicine (ACSM) recently introduced a revised model for exercise preparticipation health screening, considering three key factors: (1) an individual's current level of physical activity, (2) the presence of symptoms or diagnosed cardiovascular, metabolic, or renal disease, and (3) the intended exercise intensity. These factors help assess the risk of exercise-related cardiovascular events. Notably, the ACSM has removed risk factor assessment from this screening process. However, they recommend that individuals with diabetes who are currently inactive seek medical clearance before beginning any level of physical activity, even at low intensity [65].

While physical activity does present some risks for individuals with diabetes, such as potential acute complications including cardiac events, hypoglycemia, and hyperglycemia, the likelihood of exercise-induced adverse events is low for adults with type 2 diabetes engaging in low- to moderate-intensity activities. For individuals with type 1 diabetes, hypoglycemia is the most common exercise-related issue. Current evidence does not support the need for additional screening beyond routine diabetes care to reduce the risk of exercise-induced adverse events in asymptomatic individuals. As a result, medical clearance before exercise is unnecessary for those who are asymptomatic and receiving standard diabetes care, provided they engage in activities that do not exceed the physical demands of brisk walking or daily tasks [66, 67].

However, individuals who plan to increase exercise intensity or who meet higher-risk criteria may benefit from consulting a healthcare provider for an evaluation and possibly an exercise stress test before starting more strenuous activities. Additionally, most adults with diabetes may find it helpful to work with an exercise physiologist or a certified fitness professional with expertise in diabetes to develop a safe and effective exercise plan. Ultimately, determining an individual's risk of acute complications and selecting appropriate physical activities should be based on a thorough assessment of multiple factors, clinical judgment, and a review of their medical history and physical condition [2].

4. Aerobic exercise guidelines

Individuals with diabetes should engage in regular aerobic exercise. Ideally, each aerobic session should last at least 10 minutes, aiming for approximately 30 minutes per day on most days of the week for adults with type 2 diabetes. To reduce insulin resistance, daily exercise is encouraged, or at a minimum, no more than two consecutive days should be skipped, regardless of diabetes type. Over time, individuals should gradually increase the intensity, frequency, or duration of their workouts to reach at least 150 minutes per week of moderate-intensity exercise. Those capable of running at a speed of 6 miles per hour (9.7 km/h) for at least 25 minutes may achieve sufficient benefits with 75 minutes of vigorous-intensity exercise per week. However, since many adults, particularly those with type 2 diabetes, may find vigorous exercise too challenging, moderate-intensity exercise for the recommended duration is advised [68].

Children and adolescents with type 1 or type 2 diabetes should adhere to general physical activity guidelines for their age group. These guidelines recommend at least 60 minutes of moderate- to vigorous-intensity aerobic activity daily, along with muscle-strengthening and bone-strengthening exercises at least 3 days per week [69].

Low-volume high-intensity interval training (HIIT), which consists of short bursts of very intense exercise interspersed with longer periods of low- to moderate-intensity recovery, is an alternative to continuous aerobic exercise [6]. Recently, a 12-week HIIT program has been suggested as an effective training approach for improving serum omentin-1 levels, body composition, lipid profile, and insulin sensitivity in obese men with diabetes [70].

4.1 Resistance exercise guidelines

Adults with diabetes should engage in strength training two to three times per week on nonconsecutive days. Although heavier resistance training may provide greater benefits for glucose control and muscle strength, any form of resistance exercise is beneficial for maintaining overall physical function and balance [71].

4.2 Flexibility, balance, and other activities

Flexibility exercises should be performed at least twice a week to maintain joint mobility, but they should not replace aerobic or resistance training since they do not significantly impact glucose control [3]. Older adults, particularly those with peripheral neuropathy, should focus on balance training two to three times per week [3, 12]. Many lower-body and core exercises naturally improve balance, and activities like yoga and tai chi can be incorporated based on personal preferences.

4.3 Daily physical activity and lifestyle integration

Engaging in unstructured physical activities, such as household chores, walking, and gardening, increases energy expenditure and supports weight management. Reducing sedentary time, even in short bouts, improves post-meal glucose levels and overall glycemic control in individuals with diabetes or prediabetes. Encouraging increased daily movement is particularly beneficial for those who are sedentary and hesitant to engage in structured exercise programs [2].

4.4 Exercise timing in relation to the time of day and meals

Recent research has focused on the optimal timing of exercise for better plasma glucose control. Both the time of day and whether exercise is performed before or after meals play a crucial role in managing long-term glucose levels and post-meal plasma glucose spikes. Since the body's internal clock influences glucose regulation, it is important to consider circadian rhythms when determining the best time for physical activity. Various physiological functions, such as body temperature, glucose tolerance, insulin levels, and hormones like adiponectin and leptin, follow daily cycles. Generally, these processes function more efficiently in the morning than in the afternoon or evening in healthy individuals [72]. Some studies suggest that consuming smaller meals, especially in the evening, may improve glucose control the following day compared to large dinners (over 30% of total daily calorie intake) [49].

People with type 2 diabetes (T2D) experience circadian disruptions, with insulin sensitivity being relatively higher in the evening but decreasing overnight, leading to elevated morning glucose levels (known as the dawn phenomenon) [73]. Exercise may help realign these disrupted rhythms, though more research is needed to determine its precise effects on T2D. The natural daily fluctuations in glucose metabolism indicate that certain times of the day may be more favorable for exercise in terms of improving plasma glucose control. While some studies [74–76] indicate that exercising in the afternoon or evening is more effective for improving glucose regulation and insulin sensitivity—regardless of insulin use—others [77, 78] have found no significant differences between morning and later workouts. However, when it comes to weight management and adherence to exercise routines, morning workouts appear to be more beneficial [77]. This suggests that the ideal time for exercise depends on the desired outcome. Ultimately, the most important factor is ensuring consistency, as regular physical activity—regardless of timing—has been linked to lower mortality rates in both men and women, according to an analysis of the National Health and Nutrition Examination Survey (NHANES) [79].

Post-meal plasma glucose levels are a stronger predictor of future cardiovascular disease (CVD) risk than fasting glucose [80]. Therefore, another key question is whether it is more effective to exercise before or after eating. Engaging in physical activity after meals may enhance vascular health by reducing endothelial dysfunction and oxidative stress linked to post-meal glucose spikes [81]. However, there is limited research comparing the effects of exercising in a fasted versus fed state in people with T2D. A position statement from the American College of Sports Medicine (ACSM) concluded that post-meal exercise generally leads to better glucose control by reducing acute plasma glucose spikes, regardless of exercise type or intensity, with durations of 45 minutes or more showing the most consistent benefits [39].

A few studies have explored the impact of brief, high-intensity workouts before meals. For instance, one study found that performing six one-minute bursts of intense incline walking (at 90% maximum heart rate) 30 minutes before a meal lowered post-meal plasma glucose levels after breakfast and dinner in individuals with T2D or insulin resistance, compared to a traditional 30-minute moderate-intensity workout [82]. Another study found that cycling at moderate intensity for 60 minutes before carbohydrate intake improved insulin sensitivity and reduced insulin and lipid levels but did not significantly impact blood glucose [83]. Research has shown that short bouts of exercise after meals can help reduce glucose spikes. Examples of such exercises include: (a) three sets of one-minute light jogging with 30-second rest intervals, totaling 4 minutes per session, repeated every 30 minutes throughout the day for a total of 20 sessions; (b) three 15-minute bouts of activity at 3 metabolic equivalents (METs) after a meal [84]; (c) resistance exercises using up to 40% of body mass [85]; (d) 10 rounds of one-minute high-intensity intervals (working at 95–120% of peak power output) with one-minute low-intensity cycling between sets [75]; and (e) four intervals of three-minute exercises at approximately 56.5 ± 3.9% VO2max after breakfast [86].

Additionally, post-meal exercise has been found to lower acute serum triacylglycerol spikes following high-fat meals and mitigate the negative effects of lipid-induced oxidative stress. These benefits suggest that engaging in brief physical activity after eating may help regulate both glucose and lipid levels, ultimately supporting cardiovascular health. Collectively, these findings indicate that "exercise desserts" immediately after meals may be an effective strategy for reducing postprandial plasma glucose fluctuations [36].

5. Supervised vs. unsupervised training

Supervised exercise programs result in greater improvements in A1C, body composition, fitness, and cardiovascular health compared to unsupervised activity [24].

While unsupervised exercise can still be beneficial, it is most effective when combined with dietary interventions. Therefore, whenever feasible, supervised training is recommended for adults with diabetes to maximize health benefits [87].

Conclusion: Both aerobic and resistance training enhance insulin action, at least in the short term, and can aid in managing blood glucose levels, lipids, blood pressure, cardiovascular risk, mortality, and overall quality of life. However, to sustain these benefits, exercise must be performed consistently and should ideally incorporate a variety of training types.

Conflict of interest

The authors declare no conflict of interest.

Author details

Ahmed Ahmed[1,2]* and Samah Ismail[1,3]

1 Cairo University, Cairo, Egypt

2 Prince Sattam Bin Abdulaziz University, Al-Kharj, Saudi Arabia

3 Taibah University, Madinah, Saudi Arabia

*Address all correspondence to: ahmedaseil@yahoo.com

References

[1] Colberg SR, Sigal RJ, Fernhall B, Regensteiner JG, Blissmer BJ, Rubin RR, et al. Exercise and type 2 diabetes: The American College of Sports Medicine and the American Diabetes Association: Joint position statement. Diabetes Care. 2010;**33**(12):e147-e167

[2] Colberg SR, Sigal RJ, Yardley JE, Riddell MC, Dunstan DW, Dempsey PC, et al. Physical activity/exercise and diabetes: A position statement of the American Diabetes Association. Diabetes Care. 2016;**39**(11):2065

[3] Garber CE, Blissmer B, Deschenes MR, Franklin BA, Lamonte MJ, Lee IM, et al. Quantity and quality of exercise for developing and maintaining cardiorespiratory, musculoskeletal, and neuromotor fitness in apparently healthy adults: Guidance for prescribing exercise. Medicine and Science in Sports and Exercise. 2011;**43**(7):1334-1359

[4] Sluik D, Buijsse B, Muckelbauer R, Kaaks R, Teucher B, Tj A, et al. Physical activity and mortality in individuals with diabetes mellitus: A prospective study and meta-analysis. Archives of Internal Medicine. 2012;**172**(17):1285-1295

[5] Snowling NJ, Hopkins WG. Effects of different modes of exercise training on glucose control and risk factors for complications in type 2 diabetic patients: A meta-analysis. Diabetes Care. 2006;**29**(11):2518-2527

[6] Jelleyman C, Yates T, O'Donovan G, Gray LJ, King JA, Khunti K, et al. The effects of high-intensity interval training on glucose regulation and insulin resistance: A meta-analysis. Obesity Reviews. 2015;**16**(11):942-961

[7] Nishitani M, Shimada K, Sunayama S, Masaki Y, Kume A, Fukao K, et al. Impact of diabetes on muscle mass, muscle strength, and exercise tolerance in patients after coronary artery bypass grafting. Journal of Cardiology. 2011;**58**(2):173-180

[8] Anton SD, Karabetian C, Naugle K, Buford TW. Obesity and diabetes as accelerators of functional decline: Can lifestyle interventions maintain functional status in high risk older adults? Experimental Gerontology. 2013;**48**(9):888-897

[9] Gordon BA, Benson AC, Bird SR, Fraser SF. Resistance training improves metabolic health in type 2 diabetes: A systematic review. Diabetes Research and Clinical Practice. 2009;**83**(2):157-175

[10] Abate M, Schiavone C, Pelotti P, Salini V. Limited joint mobility in diabetes and ageing: Recent advances in pathogenesis and therapy. International Journal of Immunopathology and Pharmacology. 2010;**23**(4):997-1003

[11] Herriot MT, Colberg SR, Parson HK, Nunnold T, Vinik AI. Effects of 8 weeks of flexibility and resistance training in older adults with type 2 diabetes. Diabetes Care. 2004;**27**(12):2988-2989

[12] Morrison S, Colberg SR, Mariano M, Parson HK, Vinik AI. Balance training reduces falls risk in older individuals with type 2 diabetes. Diabetes Care. 2010;**33**(4):748-750

[13] Gillespie LD, Robertson MC, Gillespie WJ, Sherrington C, Gates S, Clemson L, et al. Interventions for preventing falls in older people living in the community. Cochrane Database of Systematic Reviews. 2012;**9**:CD007146

[14] Ahn S, Song R. Effects of tai chi exercise on glucose control, neuropathy scores, balance, and quality of life in patients with type 2 diabetes and neuropathy. The Journal of Alternative and Complementary Medicine. 2012;**18**(12):1172-1178

[15] Mikines KJ, Sonne B, Farrell PA, Tronier B, Galbo H. Effect of physical exercise on sensitivity and responsiveness to insulin in humans. American Journal of Physiology-Endocrinology and Metabolism. 1988;**254**(3):E248-E259

[16] King DS, Baldus PJ, Sharp RL, Kesl LD, Feltmeyer TL, Riddle MS. Time course for exercise-induced alterations in insulin action and glucose tolerance in middle-aged people. Journal of Applied Physiology. 1995;**78**(1):17-22

[17] Solomon TPJ, Malin SK, Karstoft K, Kashyap SR, Haus JM, Kirwan JP. Pancreatic β-cell function is a stronger predictor of changes in glycemic control after an aerobic exercise intervention than insulin sensitivity. The Journal of Clinical Endocrinology and Metabolism. 2013;**98**(10):4176-4186

[18] Hawley JA, Lessard SJ. Exercise training-induced improvements in insulin action. Acta Physiologica. 2008;**192**(1):127-135

[19] Kadoglou NPE, Iliadis F, Angelopoulou N, Perrea D, Ampatzidis G, Liapis CD, et al. The anti-inflammatory effects of exercise training in patients with type 2 diabetes mellitus. European Journal of Preventive Cardiology. 2007;**14**(6):837-843

[20] Taheri S, Zaghloul H, Chagoury O, Elhadad S, Ahmed SH, El Khatib N, et al. Effect of intensive lifestyle intervention on bodyweight and glycaemia in early type 2 diabetes (DIADEM-I): An open-label, parallel-group, randomised controlled trial. The Lancet Diabetes and Endocrinology. 2020;**8**(6):477-489

[21] Najafipour F, Mobasseri M, Yavari A, Nadrian H, Aliasgarzadeh A, Abbasi NM, et al. Effect of regular exercise training on changes in HbA1c, BMI and VO2max among patients with type 2 diabetes mellitus: An 8-year trial. BMJ Open Diabetes Research & Care. 2017;**5**(1):e000414

[22] Boulé NG, Haddad E, Kenny GP, Wells GA, Sigal RJ. Effects of exercise on glycemic control and body mass in type 2 diabetes mellitus: A meta-analysis of controlled clinical trials. Journal of the American Medical Association. 2001;**286**(10):1218-1227

[23] MacLeod SF, Terada T, Chahal BS, Boule NG. Exercise lowers postprandial glucose but not fasting glucose in type 2 diabetes: A meta-analysis of studies using continuous glucose monitoring. Diabetes/Metabolism Research and Reviews. 2013;**29**(8):593-603

[24] Umpierre D, Ribeiro PAB, Kramer CK, Leitao CB, Zucatti ATN, Azevedo MJ, et al. Physical activity advice only or structured exercise training and association with HbA1c levels in type 2 diabetes: A systematic review and meta-analysis. Journal of the American Medical Association. 2011;**305**(17):1790-1799

[25] Savikj M, Zierath JR. Train like an athlete: Applying exercise interventions to manage type 2 diabetes. Diabetologia. 2020;**63**(8):1491-1499

[26] Qadir R, Sculthorpe NF, Todd T, Brown EC. Effectiveness of resistance training and associated program characteristics in patients at risk for type 2 diabetes: A systematic review and meta-analysis. Sports Medicine-Open. 2021;**7**(1):38

[27] Dunstan DW, Daly RM, Owen N, Jolley D, De Courten M, Shaw J, et al. High-intensity resistance training improves glycemic control in older patients with type 2 diabetes. Diabetes Care. 2002;**25**(10):1729-1736

[28] Balducci S, Leonetti F, Di Mario U, Fallucca F. Is a long-term aerobic plus resistance training program feasible for and effective on metabolic profiles in type 2 diabetic patients? Diabetes Care. 2004;**27**(3):841-842

[29] Schwingshackl L, Missbach B, Dias S, König J, Hoffmann G. Impact of different training modalities on glycaemic control and blood lipids in patients with type 2 diabetes: A systematic review and network meta-analysis. Diabetologia. 2014;**57**(9):1789-1797

[30] Sigal RJ, Kenny GP, Boulé NG, Wells GA, Prud'homme D, Fortier M, et al. Effects of aerobic training, resistance training, or both on glycemic control in type 2 diabetes: A randomized trial. Annals of Internal Medicine. 2007;**147**(6):357-369

[31] Church TS, Blair SN, Cocreham S, Johannsen N, Johnson W, Kramer K, et al. Effects of aerobic and resistance training on hemoglobin A1c levels in patients with type 2 diabetes: A randomized controlled trial. Journal of the American Medical Association. 2010;**304**(20):2253-2262

[32] Balducci S, Zanuso S, Cardelli P, Salvi L, Bazuro A, Pugliese L, et al. Effect of high-versus low-intensity supervised aerobic and resistance training on modifiable cardiovascular risk factors in type 2 diabetes; the Italian diabetes and exercise study (IDES). PLoS One. 2012;**7**(11):e49297

[33] Fealy CE, Nieuwoudt S, Foucher JA, Scelsi AR, Malin SK, Pagadala M, et al. Functional high-intensity exercise training ameliorates insulin resistance and cardiometabolic risk factors in type 2 diabetes. Experimental Physiology. 2018;**103**(7):985-994

[34] Ryan AJ, Ciaraldi TP, Henry RR. Myokine regulation of insulin secretion: Impact of inflammation and type 2 diabetes. Frontiers in Physiology. 2020;**22**:10

[35] Buse JB, Ginsberg HN, Bakris GL, Clark NG, Costa F, Eckel R, et al. Primary prevention of cardiovascular diseases in people with diabetes mellitus: A scientific statement from the American Heart Association and the American Diabetes Association. Circulation. 2007;**115**:114-126

[36] Syeda USA, Battillo D, Visaria A, Malin SK. The importance of exercise for glycemic control in type 2 diabetes. American Journal of Medicine Open [Internet]. 2023;**9**:100031. Available from: https://www.sciencedirect.com/science/article/pii/S2667036423000018

[37] Trost SG. Correlates of adult's participation in physical activity: Review and update. Medicine and Science in Sports and Exercise. 2002;**34**:1996-2001

[38] Thum JS, Parsons G, Whittle T, Astorino TA. High-intensity interval training elicits higher enjoyment than moderate intensity continuous exercise. PLoS One. 2017;**12**(1):e0166299

[39] Kanaley JA, Colberg SR, Corcoran MH, Malin SK, Rodriguez NR, Crespo CJ, et al. Exercise/physical activity in individuals with type 2 diabetes: A consensus statement from the American College of Sports Medicine. Medicine and Science in Sports and Exercise. 2022;**54**(2):353

[40] Francois ME, Little JP. Effectiveness and safety of high-intensity interval training in patients with type 2 diabetes. Diabetes Spectrum: A Publication of the American Diabetes Association. 2015;**28**(1):39

[41] Little JP, Gillen JB, Percival ME, Safdar A, Tarnopolsky MA, Punthakee Z, et al. Low-volume high-intensity interval training reduces hyperglycemia and increases muscle mitochondrial capacity in patients with type 2 diabetes. Journal of Applied Physiology. 2011;**111**(6):1554-1560

[42] Madsen SM, Thorup AC, Overgaard K, Jeppesen PB. High intensity interval training improves glycaemic control and pancreatic β cell function of type 2 diabetes patients. PLoS One. 2015;**10**(8):e0133286

[43] Grace A, Chan E, Giallauria F, Graham PL, Smart NA. Clinical outcomes and glycaemic responses to different aerobic exercise training intensities in type II diabetes: A systematic review and meta-analysis. Cardiovascular Diabetology. 2017;**16**:1-10

[44] de Matos MA, Vieira DV, Pinhal KC, Lopes JF, Dias-Peixoto MF, Pauli JR, et al. High-intensity interval training improves markers of oxidative metabolism in skeletal muscle of individuals with obesity and insulin resistance. Frontiers in Physiology. 2018;**9**:1451

[45] Winding KM, Munch GW, Iepsen UW, Van Hall G, Pedersen BK, Mortensen SP. The effect on glycaemic control of low-volume high-intensity interval training versus endurance training in individuals with type 2 diabetes. Diabetes, Obesity & Metabolism. 2018;**20**(5):1131-1139

[46] Xin LJ, Zhu L, Jun LP, Li N, Bing XY. Effectiveness of high-intensity interval training on glycemic control and cardiorespiratory fitness in patients with type 2 diabetes: A systematic review and meta-analysis. Aging Clinical and Experimental Research. 2019;**31**:575-593

[47] Way KL, Sabag A, Sultana RN, Baker MK, Keating SE, Lanting S, et al. The effect of low-volume high-intensity interval training on cardiovascular health outcomes in type 2 diabetes: A randomised controlled trial. International Journal of Cardiology. 2020;**320**:148-154

[48] Qiu S, Cai X, Yin H, Sun Z, Zügel M, Steinacker JM, et al. Exercise training and endothelial function in patients with type 2 diabetes: A meta-analysis. Cardiovascular Diabetology. 2018;**17**:1-12

[49] Magalhães JP, Melo X, Correia IR, Ribeiro RT, Raposo J, Dores H, et al. Effects of combined training with different intensities on vascular health in patients with type 2 diabetes: A 1-year randomized controlled trial. Cardiovascular Diabetology. 2019;**18**:1-13

[50] Roberts CK, Hevener AL, Barnard RJ. Metabolic syndrome and insulin resistance: Underlying causes and modification by exercise training. Comprehensive Physiology. 2013;**3**(1):1

[51] Magkos F, Tsekouras Y, Kavouras SA, Mittendorfer B, Sidossis LS. Improved insulin sensitivity after a single bout of exercise is curvilinearly related to exercise energy expenditure. Clinical Science. 2008;**114**(1):59-64

[52] Wojtaszewski JFP, Nielsen JN, Richter EA. Invited review: Effect of acute exercise on insulin signaling and action in humans. Journal of Applied Physiology. 2002;**93**(1):384-392

[53] Wang X, Patterson BW, Smith GI, Kampelman J, Reeds DN, Sullivan SA,

et al. A~ 60-min brisk walk increases insulin-stimulated glucose disposal but has no effect on hepatic and adipose tissue insulin sensitivity in older women. Journal of Applied Physiology. 2013;**114**(11):1563-1568

[54] Gillen JB, Little JP, Punthakee Z, Tarnopolsky MA, Riddell MC, Gibala MJ. Acute high-intensity interval exercise reduces the postprandial glucose response and prevalence of hyperglycaemia in patients with type 2 diabetes. Diabetes, Obesity & Metabolism. 2012;**14**(6):575-577

[55] Manders RJ, Van Dijk JW, Van Loon LJ. Low-intensity exercise reduces the prevalence of hyperglycemia in type 2 diabetes. Medicine and Science in Sports and Exercise. 2010;**42**(2):219-225

[56] Newsom SA, Everett AC, Hinko A, Horowitz JF. A single session of low-intensity exercise is sufficient to enhance insulin sensitivity into the next day in obese adults. Diabetes Care. 2013;**36**(9):2516-2522

[57] Bacchi E, Negri C, Targher G, Faccioli N, Lanza M, Zoppini G, et al. Both resistance training and aerobic training reduce hepatic fat content in type 2 diabetic subjects with nonalcoholic fatty liver disease (the RAED2 randomized trial). Hepatology. 2013;**58**(4):1287-1295

[58] Hallsworth K, Fattakhova G, Hollingsworth KG, Thoma C, Moore S, Taylor R, et al. Resistance exercise reduces liver fat and its mediators in non-alcoholic fatty liver disease independent of weight loss. Gut. 2011;**60**(9):1278-1283

[59] Kirwan JP, Solomon TPJ, Wojta DM, Staten MA, Holloszy JO. Effects of 7 days of exercise training on insulin sensitivity and responsiveness in type 2 diabetes mellitus. American Journal of Physiology-Endocrinology and Metabolism. 2009;**297**(1):E151-E156

[60] Dubé JJ, Fleishman K, Rousson V, Goodpaster BH, Amati F. Exercise dose and insulin sensitivity: Relevance for diabetes prevention. Medicine and Science in Sports and Exercise. 2012;**44**(5):793

[61] Lin X, Zhang X, Guo J, Roberts CK, McKenzie S, Wu W, et al. Effects of exercise training on cardiorespiratory fitness and biomarkers of cardiometabolic health: A systematic review and meta-analysis of randomized controlled trials. Journal of the American Heart Association. 2015;**4**(7):e002014

[62] Wing RR, Bolin P, Brancati FL, Bray GA, Clark JM, Coday M, et al. Cardiovascular effects of intensive lifestyle intervention in type 2 diabetes. Diabetes Technology & Therapeutics. 2014;**16**(Suppl. 1):S97-S98

[63] Pi-Sunyer X. The look AHEAD trial: A review and discussion of its outcomes. Current Nutrition Reports. 2014;**3**:387-391

[64] Yang Z, Scott CA, Mao C, Tang J, Farmer AJ. Resistance exercise versus aerobic exercise for type 2 diabetes: A systematic review and meta-analysis. Sports Medicine. 2014;**44**:487-499

[65] Riebe D, Franklin BA, Thompson PD, Garber CE, Whitfield GP, Magal M, et al. Updating ACSM's recommendations for exercise preparticipation health screening. Medicine and Science in Sports and Exercise. 2015;**47**(11):2473-2479

[66] Young LH, Frans J, Chyun DA, Davey JA, Barrett EJ, Taillefer R, et al. Cardiac outcomes after screening for asymptomatic coronary

artery disease in patients with type 2 diabetes: The DIAD study: A randomized controlled trial. Journal of the American Medical Association. 2009;**301**(15):1547-1555

[67] Lièvre MM, Moulin P, Thivolet C, Rodier M, Rigalleau V, Penfornis A, et al. Detection of silent myocardial ischemia in asymptomatic patients with diabetes: Results of a randomized trial and meta-analysis assessing the effectiveness of systematic screening. Trials. 2011;**12**:1-7

[68] Tonoli C, Heyman E, Roelands B, Buyse L, Cheung SS, Berthoin S, et al. Effects of different types of acute and chronic (training) exercise on glycaemic control in type 1 diabetes mellitus: A meta-analysis. Sports Medicine. 2012;**42**:1059-1080

[69] Buchner DM. Physical activity and prevention of cardiovascular disease in older adults. Clinics in Geriatric Medicine. 2009;**25**(4):661-675

[70] Ahmed AS, Ahmed MS. The impact of high intensity interval training on serum omentin-1 levels, lipid profile, and insulin resistance in obese men with type 2 diabetes mellitus. Isokinetics and Exercise Science. 2023;**31**(3):221-231

[71] Willey KA, Singh MAF. Battling insulin resistance in elderly obese people with type 2 diabetes: Bring on the heavy weights. Diabetes Care. 2003;**26**(5):1580-1588

[72] Mancilla R, Krook A, Schrauwen P, Hesselink MKC. Diurnal regulation of peripheral glucose metabolism: Potential effects of exercise timing. Obesity. 2020;**28**:S38-S45

[73] Heden TD, Kanaley JA. Syncing exercise with meals and circadian clocks. Exercise and Sport Sciences Reviews. 2019;**47**(1):22-28

[74] Hetherington-Rauth M, Magalhães JP, Rosa GB, Correia IR, Carneiro T, Oliveira EC, et al. Morning versus afternoon physical activity and health-related outcomes in individuals with type 2 diabetes. Diabetes, Obesity & Metabolism. 2022;**24**(6):1172-1175

[75] Savikj M, Gabriel BM, Alm PS, Smith J, Caidahl K, Björnholm M, et al. Afternoon exercise is more efficacious than morning exercise at improving blood glucose levels in individuals with type 2 diabetes: A randomised crossover trial. Diabetologia. 2019;**62**:233-237

[76] Moholdt T, Parr EB, Devlin BL, Debik J, Giskeødegård G, Hawley JA. The effect of morning vs evening exercise training on glycaemic control and serum metabolites in overweight/obese men: A randomised trial. Diabetologia. 2021;**64**(9):2061-2076

[77] Schumacher LM, Thomas JG, Raynor HA, Rhodes RE, Bond DS. Consistent morning exercise may be beneficial for individuals with obesity. Exercise and Sport Sciences Reviews. 2020;**48**(4):201-208

[78] Teo SYM, Kanaley JA, Guelfi KJ, Marston KJ, Fairchild TJ. The impact of exercise timing on glycemic control: A randomized clinical trial. Medicine and Science in Sports and Exercise. 2020;**52**(2):323-334

[79] Ma T, Xie YJ, Bennett T, Lee CD. Time-of-day moderate-to-vigorous physical activity and all-cause mortality in individuals with type 2 diabetes. Journal of Sports Sciences. 2022;**40**(6):614-620

[80] Hershon KS, Hirsch BR, Odugbesan O. Importance of postprandial glucose in relation to A1C and cardiovascular disease. Clinical Diabetes. 2019;**37**(3):250-259

[81] Adamovich Y, Dandavate V, Ezagouri S, Manella G, Zwighaft Z, Sobel J, et al. Clock proteins and training modify exercise capacity in a daytime-dependent manner. National Academy of Sciences of the United States of America. 2021;**118**(35):e2101115118

[82] Francois ME, Baldi JC, Manning PJ, Lucas SJE, Hawley JA, Williams MJA, et al. 'Exercise snacks' before meals: A novel strategy to improve glycaemic control in individuals with insulin resistance. Diabetologia. 2014;**57**(7):1437-1445

[83] Edinburgh RM, Bradley HE, Abdullah NF, Robinson SL, Chrzanowski-Smith OJ, Walhin JP, et al. Lipid metabolism links nutrient-exercise timing to insulin sensitivity in men classified as overweight or obese. The Journal of Clinical Endocrinology and Metabolism. 2020;**105**(3):660-676

[84] DiPietro L, Gribok A, Stevens MS, Hamm LF, Rumpler W. Three 15-min bouts of moderate postmeal walking significantly improves 24-h glycemic control in older people at risk for impaired glucose tolerance. Diabetes Care. 2013;**36**(10):3262-3268

[85] Heden TD, Winn NC, Mari A, Booth FW, Rector RS, Thyfault JP, et al. Postdinner resistance exercise improves postprandial risk factors more effectively than predinner resistance exercise in patients with type 2 diabetes. Journal of Applied Physiology. 2015;**118**(5):624-634

[86] Larsen JJS, Dela F, Madsbad S, Galbo H. The effect of intense exercise on postprandial glucose homeostasis in type II diabetic patients. Diabetologia. 1999;**42**:1282-1292

[87] Balducci S, Zanuso S, Nicolucci A, De Feo P, Cavallo S, Cardelli P, et al. Effect of an intensive exercise intervention strategy on modifiable cardiovascular risk factors in subjects with type 2 diabetes mellitus: A randomized controlled trial: The Italian diabetes and exercise study (IDES). Archives of Internal Medicine. 2010;**170**(20):1794-1803

Chapter 4

New and Interesting Benefits with New Molecules in Obesity and Type 2 Diabetes

Fernando Grover Páez, Sofía Zubieta Barrios, Luz Elena Cortes Bautista, Luis Diego Pantoja Chong and Ximena Guadalupe Reynoso Velazquez

Abstract

Glucagon-like peptide-1 receptor agonists (GLP-1 RAs) are highly effective therapies for managing type 2 diabetes mellitus (T2DM) and obesity. These agents mimic the incretin hormone GLP-1, enhancing glucose-dependent insulin secretion, suppressing glucagon release, delaying gastric emptying, and promoting satiety. Mechanistically, GLP-1 RAs target the GLP-1 receptor, predominantly found in pancreatic β-cells, the gastrointestinal tract, and the central nervous system, leading to improved glycemic control with a reduced risk of hypoglycemia. Their weight-loss benefits stem from delayed gastric emptying and central appetite suppression, while cardiovascular benefits, such as reduced major adverse cardiovascular events, make them integral to T2DM treatment. GLP-1 RAs differ in pharmacokinetics, with short-acting agents, like exenatide, targeting postprandial glucose, and long-acting options, like liraglutide and semaglutide, offering sustained fasting and postprandial glucose control. Semaglutide, available as both injectable and oral formulations, has demonstrated superior efficacy in weight reduction and glycemic outcomes compared to its counterparts. Additionally, emerging dual and triple agonists targeting GLP-1, glucose-dependent insulinotropic polypeptide (GIP), and glucagon receptors, such as tirzepatide, represent a novel therapeutic frontier, amplifying metabolic benefits with substantial weight loss and improved glycemic control. While GLP-1 RAs are generally well-tolerated, gastrointestinal side effects, such as nausea and vomiting, remain the most common adverse events. Long-term safety, particularly concerning pancreatitis and gallbladder disease, requires further study. Nonetheless, their efficacy and safety profiles solidify their role as cornerstone therapies for metabolic diseases. Ongoing advancements in multi-agonist therapies promise enhanced therapeutic outcomes and broader clinical utility in the management of T2DM and obesity.

Keywords: GLP-1 receptor agonists, incretin-based therapy, glycemic control, weight loss, dual and triple agonists, tirzepatide, retatrutide, survodutide

1. Introduction

Glucagon-like peptide-1 receptor agonists (GLP-1) RAs exert their effects by mimicking the incretin hormone GLP-1, enhancing glucose-dependent insulin secretion, suppressing glucagon release, delaying gastric emptying, and promoting satiety (**Figure 1**). This unique pharmacological profile has positioned GLP-1 RAs as dual-purpose agents for glycemic control and weight reduction, offering substantial benefits for patients with obesity and T2DM. Clinical trials and meta-analyses consistently demonstrate the efficacy of GLP-1 RAs in achieving significant weight loss and improved glycemic outcomes, often surpassing traditional therapeutic agents for diabetes management. For instance, high-dose GLP-1 RAs, such as liraglutide and semaglutide, have been shown to induce clinically meaningful reductions in body weight and hemoglobin A1c (HbA1c), with additional benefits in cardiovascular risk reduction [1, 2].

Recent advances in GLP-1 receptor pharmacology have further expanded the therapeutic potential of these agents. Studies investigating their use in higher doses, extended formulations, and as part of dual- or triple-agonist therapies have revealed unprecedented outcomes in managing obesity and its comorbidities. The introduction of dual GLP-1/glucose-dependent insulinotropic polypeptide (GIP) receptor agonists, such as tirzepatide, represents a paradigm shift, combining the benefits of GLP-1 RAs with additional anti-inflammatory and vascular protective properties attributed to GIP signaling, [3–5] and recently Survodutide (BI 456906), has arisen as a novel subcutaneous GCGR/GLP-1R dual agonist in development for the treatment of people with type 2 diabetes, obesity and non-alcoholic steatohepatitis (NASH) [6].

The increasing prevalence of obesity and diabetes needs a comprehensive exploration of therapies that address not only glycemic control but also metabolic and cardiovascular risk factors. This chapter provides an in-depth examination of the role of GLP-1 RAs in the treatment of obesity and T2DM, emphasizing the evidence-based benefits and emerging trends in the use of these pharmacological agents. The integration of GLP-1 RAs into clinical practice highlights their potential to redefine the therapeutic landscape for patients struggling with obesity-related metabolic disorders.

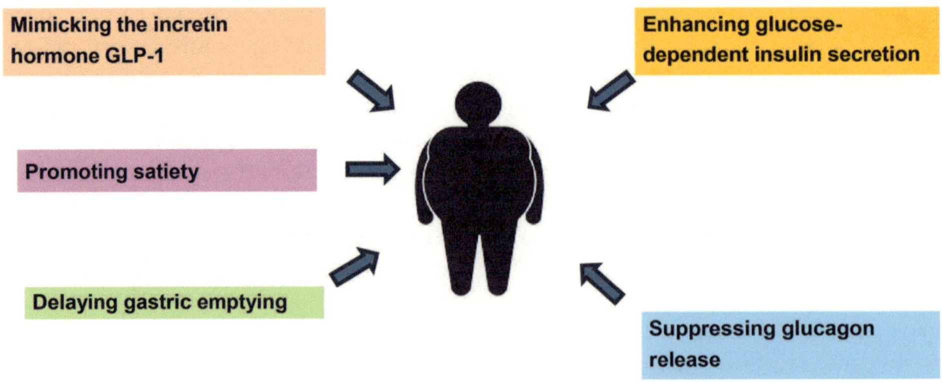

Figure 1.
Effects GLP-1 RAs.

DOI: http://dx.doi.org/10.5772/intechopen.1009256

2. Pathophysiology of obesity

Obesity remains a global health challenge, with its prevalence escalating over recent years. Understanding its complex pathophysiology is crucial for developing effective interventions.

2.1 Genetic and epigenetic influences

Recent studies have reinforced the significant role of genetics in obesity. Monogenic forms, resulting from single-gene mutations, and polygenic obesity, involving multiple genetic variants, contribute to individual susceptibility [1, 2]. Epigenetic modifications, influenced by environmental factors, further modulate gene expression related to adiposity and metabolic regulation [3, 4]. These insights underscore the intricate interplay between genetic predisposition and environmental exposures in obesity development [5].

2.2 Adipose tissue dysfunction and inflammation

Adipose tissue is now recognized as an active endocrine organ. In obesity, adipocyte hypertrophy and hyperplasia lead to hypoxia and subsequent inflammation [7, 8]. This state is characterized by increased infiltration of immune cells, particularly macrophages, which shift from an anti-inflammatory (M2) to a pro-inflammatory (M1) phenotype. The resulting chronic low-grade inflammation disrupts adipokine secretion, notably decreasing adiponectin and increasing leptin levels, contributing to systemic insulin resistance and metabolic dysregulation [9, 10].

2.3 Neuroendocrine regulation and appetite control

The central nervous system, especially the hypothalamus, plays a pivotal role in energy homeostasis. Recent research has elucidated how dysregulation in neuroendocrine pathways affects appetite and satiety signals [10, 11]. Alterations in hormones such as ghrelin, peptide YY, and glucagon-like peptide-1 (GLP-1) have been implicated in disrupted hunger cues, promoting excessive caloric intake and weight gain [12–14].

2.4 Gut microbiota and metabolic interactions

Advancements in metagenomics have highlighted the gut microbiota's influence on obesity. Dysbiosis, or microbial imbalance, affects energy harvest from the diet and modulates inflammatory pathways. Specific microbial profiles have been associated with increased adiposity, suggesting that targeting the microbiome could offer novel therapeutic avenues for obesity management [13, 14].

2.5 Insulin resistance and metabolic complications

Obesity-induced inflammation and adipokine imbalance contribute to the development of insulin resistance. This condition impairs glucose uptake in peripheral tissues, elevating blood glucose levels and increasing the risk of type 2 diabetes mellitus (T2DM) [6, 7]. Understanding the molecular mechanisms linking obesity to

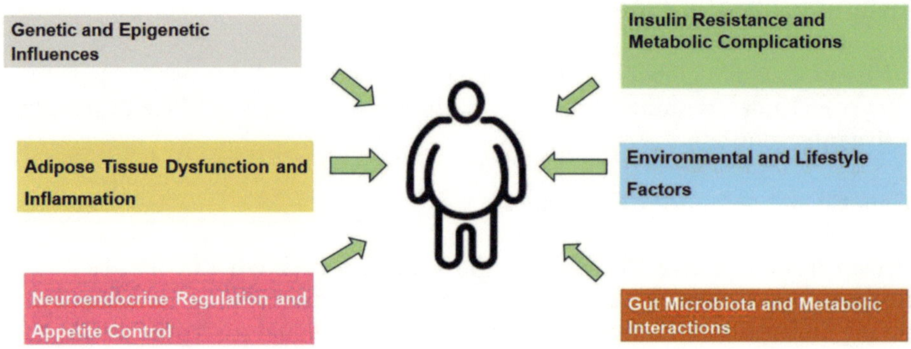

Figure 2.
Pathophysiology of obesity.

insulin resistance is essential for developing targeted treatments to mitigate associated metabolic complications [9, 10].

2.6 Environmental and lifestyle factors

Beyond biological mechanisms, environmental and lifestyle factors significantly influence obesity prevalence. Sedentary behavior, high-calorie diets, and socio-economic determinants interact with genetic predispositions, exacerbating weight gain [3, 12]. Public health strategies focusing on lifestyle modifications remain critical components in addressing the obesity epidemic (**Figure 2**) [15].

2.7 Therapeutic implications and future directions

The deepening understanding of obesity's pathophysiology has paved the way for innovative therapeutic approaches. Pharmacological agents targeting specific pathways, such as GLP-1 receptor agonists, have shown promise in weight management [16, 17]. Additionally, personalized medicine, considering individual genetic and microbiome profiles, holds potential for more effective interventions. Ongoing research is essential to translate these insights into clinical practice, aiming to curb the global obesity crisis [18–23], in conclusion, the past two years have yielded significant insights into the multifaceted pathophysiology of obesity. Integrating genetic, inflammatory, neuroendocrine, and environmental perspectives is essential for developing comprehensive strategies to combat this pervasive health issue. Continued interdisciplinary research and public health initiatives are imperative to address the complexities of obesity and its associated comorbidities [9, 13].

3. Pathophysiology of type 2 diabetes: Focus on GLP-1, GIP, and glucagon receptor agonists

T2DM is a complex metabolic disorder characterized by chronic hyperglycemia, insulin resistance, and progressive β-cell dysfunction. Recent studies have highlighted the intricate role of incretin hormones such as GLP-1, GIP, and glucagon in the regulation of glucose and energy metabolism. Therapeutic advancements targeting these pathways have transformed the management of T2DM, offering improved glycemic control, weight reduction, and cardiovascular benefits [24].

3.1 GLP-1 receptor agonists

GLP-1 RAs mimic the incretin hormone GLP-1, enhancing insulin secretion, suppressing glucagon release, delaying gastric emptying, and promoting satiety. These actions collectively improve glycemic control while addressing obesity-related complications in T2DM. Semaglutide, liraglutide, and dulaglutide are among the most studied GLP-1 RAs, demonstrating significant reductions in HbA1c and body weight in clinical trials [25–27]. Furthermore, GLP-1 RAs have shown cardiovascular protective effects, reducing the risk of major adverse cardiovascular events (MACE) in high-risk patients [28].

On the other hand, recent research has also explored higher doses and innovative delivery methods, such as oral semaglutide, to enhance patient adherence [28–30]. These advancements further cement the role of GLP-1 RAs as cornerstone therapies for T2DM management.

3.2 GIP receptor agonists

Glucose insulinotrophic peptide (GIP), another incretin hormone, stimulates insulin secretion in a glucose-dependent manner. However, its insulinotropic effect is diminished in individuals with T2DM. Novel therapies targeting GIP receptors aim to restore its regulatory role in glucose homeostasis. Studies have revealed that GIP can enhance β-cell function, particularly when combined with GLP-1 receptor activation, creating synergistic effects [29].

Dual GLP-1/GIP receptor agonists, such as tirzepatide, have emerged as groundbreaking therapies. Tirzepatide has demonstrated superior efficacy compared to GLP-1 RAs alone, achieving unprecedented reductions in HbA1c and body weight while maintaining a favorable safety profile [30].

3.3 Glucagon receptor agonists

While glucagon traditionally plays a counter-regulatory role by increasing hepatic glucose production, recent studies have identified its potential in energy expenditure and lipid metabolism. Dual GLP-1/glucagon receptor agonists, such as cotadutide, exploit these properties, combining glucagon's lipolytic effects with GLP-1-mediated glycemic control [31, 32]. This dual mechanism offers a promising approach to managing both T2DM and obesity.

Furthermore, triagonists targeting GLP-1, GIP, and glucagon receptors are under investigation, aiming to maximize metabolic benefits. Early trials have shown significant improvements in weight loss and glycemic control, suggesting a transformative potential in T2DM treatment [30].

3.4 Therapeutic implications and future directions

The integration of incretin-based therapies into clinical practice has redefined the treatment paradigm for T2DM. GLP-1, GIP, and glucagon receptor agonists not only improve glycemic control but also address obesity and cardiovascular risk factors, critical components of the T2DM disease burden [31].

Future research is focused on optimizing these therapies through dose refinement, combination regimens, and personalized medicine approaches. Additionally, understanding the long-term effects and safety profiles of these agents remains essential to their widespread adoption.

4. Pharmacology of GLP-1 receptor agonists

GLP-1 RAs are a cornerstone in the treatment of T2DM and obesity. These agents mimic the incretin hormone GLP-1, enhancing glucose-dependent insulin secretion, suppressing glucagon release, delaying gastric emptying, and promoting satiety.

4.1 Mechanism of action

GLP-1 RAs target the GLP-1 receptor, a member of the G-protein-coupled receptor family, predominantly expressed in pancreatic β-cells, the gastrointestinal tract, and the central nervous system. Activation of this receptor leads to increased intracellular cyclic AMP (cAMP), enhancing glucose-stimulated insulin secretion and suppressing glucagon release in a glucose-dependent manner. These effects improve glycemic control while minimizing the risk of hypoglycemia [32].

In addition to their pancreatic effects, GLP-1 RAs delay gastric emptying and act on hypothalamic centers to reduce appetite, contributing to weight loss. Their cardiovascular benefits, including improved endothelial function and anti-inflammatory effects, further support their role in reducing cardiovascular risks in T2DM patients [33].

4.2 Pharmacokinetics and pharmacodynamics

GLP-1 RAs vary in their pharmacokinetic properties, influencing dosing regimens and patient adherence. Short-acting agents, such as exenatide twice daily, predominantly target postprandial glucose levels due to transient receptor activation.

Long-acting agents, including liraglutide, dulaglutide, and semaglutide, provide sustained receptor activation, effectively lowering fasting and postprandial glucose levels [30].

4.3 Pharmacology of the most important GLP-1 RAs

Exenatide: A synthetic version of exendin-4 with a half-life of 2–4 hours, requiring twice-daily administration. It was the first GLP-1 RA introduced and primarily reduces postprandial glucose excursions [34].

Liraglutide: A long-acting analog with a half-life of approximately 13 hours, requiring once-daily administration. It has demonstrated cardiovascular benefits in addition to glycemic control [35].

Dulaglutide: Engineered as a fusion protein with a half-life of 5 days, allowing for once-weekly dosing. Its molecular structure reduces renal clearance and immunogenicity.

Semaglutide: Available as a weekly injection or daily oral formulation. It has shown superior efficacy in weight reduction and HbA1c control compared to other GLP-1 Ras.

Albiglutide and Lixisenatide: These agents provide alternative options with varying pharmacodynamic profiles, targeting specific patient populations [36].

4.4 Clinical efficacy

Head-to-head trials consistently demonstrate significant reductions in HbA1c (0.5–1.5%) and body weight (3–6 kg) across GLP-1 RAs, with semaglutide often showing the greatest efficacy. Cardiovascular outcome trials (CVOTs) such as LEADER and SUSTAIN-6 highlight their role in reducing MACE [35, 36].

4.5 Safety and tolerability

Gastrointestinal side effects, including nausea and vomiting, are the most common adverse events, often transient and dose-dependent. Rare but serious concerns, such as pancreatitis and gallbladder disease, require further investigation. Their favorable risk-benefit profile, however, supports widespread use [33].

4.6 Emerging trends

The development of dual and triple agonists targeting GLP-1, GIP, and glucagon receptors, such as tirzepatide, represents an exciting frontier. These agents aim to amplify metabolic benefits, achieving superior glycemic control and weight loss [37]. In conclusion, GLP-1 receptor agonists are transformative in managing T2DM and obesity. Their diverse pharmacological profiles, robust efficacy, and safety establish them as essential therapies. Ongoing innovation, particularly with multi-agonist therapies, promises to further enhance their clinical utility.

5. Pharmacology of dual GLP-1 and GIP receptor agonists

Dual agonists targeting both GLP-1 and GIP receptors represent a novel therapeutic approach in the management of T2DM and obesity. These agents, exemplified by tirzepatide, aim to harness the synergistic effects of GLP-1 and GIP to enhance glycemic control and promote weight loss.

5.1 Mechanism of action

GLP-1 and GIP are incretin hormones that play crucial roles in glucose homeostasis. GLP-1 enhances glucose-dependent insulin secretion, suppresses glucagon release, delays gastric emptying, and promotes satiety. GIP also stimulates insulin secretion in a glucose-dependent manner but has a less pronounced effect on glucagon suppression and gastric emptying. Dual agonists activate both receptors, potentially amplifying these beneficial effects. Notably, the simultaneous activation of GLP-1 and GIP receptors may lead to improved insulin sensitivity and more substantial reductions in body weight compared to GLP-1 receptor agonists alone.

5.2 Pharmacokinetics and pharmacodynamics

Tirzepatide is the most advanced dual GLP-1/GIP receptor agonist, administered as a once-weekly subcutaneous injection. It exhibits a half-life conducive to weekly dosing, facilitating patient adherence. Clinical trials have demonstrated that tirzepatide significantly reduces HbA1c levels and body weight in patients with T2DM. The pharmacodynamic profile of tirzepatide indicates enhanced insulin secretion, improved insulin sensitivity, and reduced food intake, contributing to its efficacy in glycemic control and weight management [38].

5.3 Clinical efficacy

In clinical studies, tirzepatide has shown superior efficacy in lowering HbA1c and body weight compared to existing GLP-1 receptor agonists. For instance, patients treated with tirzepatide achieved mean HbA1c reductions exceeding 2% and weight loss up to 12 kg over 40 weeks. These outcomes suggest that dual agonism may offer advantages over selective GLP-1 receptor activation, particularly in patients requiring substantial weight reduction alongside glycemic control [39, 40].

5.4 Safety and tolerability

The safety profile of dual GLP-1/GIP receptor agonists is generally consistent with that of GLP-1 receptor agonists, with gastrointestinal adverse events such as nausea, vomiting, and diarrhea being the most commonly reported side effects. These symptoms are typically transient and dose-dependent. Ongoing studies are assessing the long-term safety of these agents, including their cardiovascular outcomes and potential risks associated with chronic use [41–45].

5.5 Emerging therapies

Beyond tirzepatide, other dual agonists are under investigation. For example, CT-388 is a novel dual GLP-1 and GIP receptor modulator designed for once-weekly subcutaneous administration. Early-phase clinical trials have reported significant weight loss with CT-388, indicating its potential as an effective treatment for obesity and T2DM. In conclusion, Dual GLP-1 and GIP receptor agonists represent a significant advancement in the pharmacotherapy of T2DM and obesity. By leveraging the complementary actions of GLP-1 and GIP, these agents offer enhanced glycemic control and weight reduction compared to existing therapies. Ongoing research will further elucidate their long-term efficacy and safety profiles, potentially expanding their therapeutic applications [46].

6. Pharmacology of triple-action agonists targeting GLP-1, GIP, and glucagon receptors in the treatment of obesity and type 2 diabetes

In recent years, the development of multi-receptor agonists targeting GLP-1, GIP, and glucagon receptors has emerged as a promising therapeutic strategy for obesity and T2DM. These triple agonists aim to harness the synergistic effects of these hormones to improve glycemic control and induce weight loss [47].

6.1 Mechanism of action

Triple agonists simultaneously activate GLP-1, GIP, and glucagon receptors, leading to a multifaceted metabolic response. Activation of GLP-1 receptors enhances insulin secretion, inhibits glucagon release, slows gastric emptying, and promotes satiety. GIP receptor activation further stimulates insulin secretion and may have direct effects on adipose tissue, enhancing lipid metabolism. Glucagon receptor activation increases energy expenditure by promoting hepatic glucose production and lipolysis. The combined activation of these receptors results in improved glycemic control and significant weight reduction.

7. Recent developments

Retatrutide (LY3437943) is a novel triple agonist that shows promising results in clinical trials. In a phase 2 trial involving adults with obesity, retatrutide treatment for 48 weeks resulted in substantial reductions in body weight, with participants achieving up to 24.2% weight loss. Additionally, improvements in glycemic control were observed, indicating its potential efficacy in T2DM management.

Another study demonstrated that triple agonism of GLP-1, GIP, and glucagon receptors resulted in greater weight loss and reduction in blood glucose levels in obese mice compared to monoagonists and dual agonists. This preclinical evidence supports the therapeutic potential of triple agonists in metabolic disorders [47, 48].

7.1 Pharmacokinetics and pharmacodynamics

Triple agonists are typically administered *via* subcutaneous injection. The pharmacokinetic profiles are designed to allow for once-weekly dosing, enhancing patient compliance. These agents exhibit a balanced activity across GLP-1, GIP, and glucagon receptors, ensuring a coordinated metabolic response. The pharmacodynamic effects include enhanced insulin secretion, reduced appetite, increased energy expenditure, and improved lipid metabolism, contributing to their efficacy in obesity and T2DM treatment [48].

7.2 Safety and tolerability

The safety profile of triple agonists is generally consistent with that of GLP-1 receptor agonists. Common adverse events include gastrointestinal symptoms such as nausea, vomiting, and diarrhea, which are typically transient and diminish over time. No significant safety concerns have been reported in clinical trials to date; however, long-term studies are necessary to fully assess their safety profile. In conclusion, triple-action agonists targeting GLP-1, GIP, and glucagon receptors represent a novel and promising approach in the treatment of obesity and T2DM. The synergistic effects of these hormones offer significant advantages in terms of weight loss and glycemic control. Ongoing clinical trials and future research will further elucidate their therapeutic potential and long-term safety [49, 50].

8. Pleiotropic effects of GLP-1, GIP, and glucagon receptor agonists

GLP-1, GIP, and glucagon receptor agonists have gained attention for their therapeutic effects in obesity and T2DM. Beyond their primary roles in glycemic control, these agonists exhibit pleiotropic effects, influencing cardiovascular health, inflammation, and energy metabolism.

8.1 Cardiovascular benefits

GLP-1 receptor agonists have demonstrated cardioprotective properties in both diabetic and non-diabetic populations. These effects include reduced MACE, improved endothelial function, and decreased arterial stiffness. For example, the LEADER trial with liraglutide showed a 13% reduction in MACE among high-risk patients with T2DM [51]. Similarly, tirzepatide, a dual GIP and GLP-1 receptor agonist, has shown reductions in cardiovascular risk biomarkers, such as triglycerides and C-reactive protein, further highlighting its cardiometabolic benefit [52].

8.2 Anti-inflammatory and immune modulation

Chronic inflammation is a hallmark of obesity and T2DM, contributing to insulin resistance and cardiovascular disease. GLP-1 receptor activation has been linked to reduced levels of inflammatory markers such as interleukin-6 (IL-6) and tumor necrosis factor-alpha (TNF-α). Moreover, dual and triple agonists that incorporate GIP and glucagon receptor targeting have shown enhanced anti-inflammatory effects. For instance, tirzepatide has demonstrated superior reductions in inflammatory markers compared to GLP-1 receptor agonists alone, indicating a synergistic interaction between GIP and GLP-1 pathways [53, 54].

8.3 Effects on energy expenditure and fat metabolism

Glucagon receptor agonists play a pivotal role in increasing energy expenditure and promoting lipolysis. This complements the satiety-inducing and appetite-suppressing effects of GLP-1 and GIP receptor activation. Triple agonists such as retatrutide have shown unprecedented reductions in body weight in clinical trials, with up to 24% reductions observed in phase 2 studies. This effect is attributed to a balanced stimulation of energy expenditure, appetite suppression, and enhanced lipid metabolism [55, 56].

8.4 Renal protection

Emerging evidence suggests that GLP-1 receptor agonists may confer renoprotective effects by reducing albuminuria and preserving glomerular filtration rates (GFR). These benefits are thought to be mediated through improvements in hemodynamic regulation, reductions in oxidative stress, and anti-inflammatory actions. Dual agonists, such as tirzepatide, may amplify these effects, although long-term studies are needed to confirm these findings [57–59].

8.5 Neuroprotective effects

GLP-1 receptor agonists also exhibit potential neuroprotective benefits, including improved cognitive function and reduced neuroinflammation. Preclinical studies indicate that GLP-1 receptor activation can mitigate amyloid-beta accumulation and improve synaptic plasticity, suggesting a role in delaying neurodegenerative diseases such as Alzheimer's disease. While data on dual and triple agonists are limited, their broader metabolic effects may enhance neuroprotection (**Figure 3**) [60, 61].

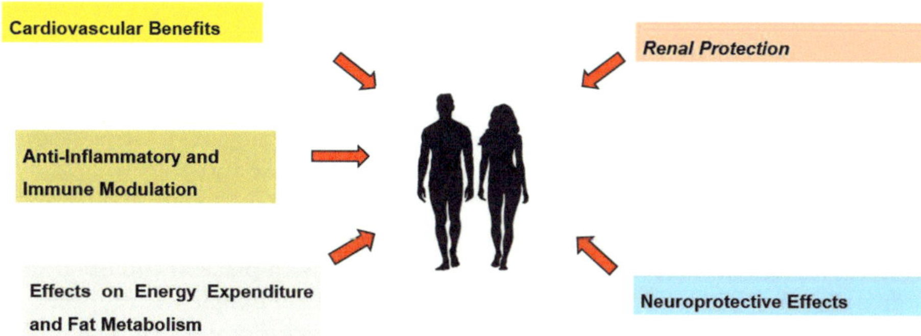

Figure 3.
Pleiotropic effects of GLP-1, GIP, and glucagon receptor agonists.

9. Conclusion

The pleiotropic effects of GLP-1, GIP, and glucagon receptor agonists extend beyond glycemic control, offering significant benefits in cardiovascular health, inflammation, energy metabolism, renal function, and neuroprotection. These agents represent a paradigm shift in the management of metabolic disorders, providing a holistic approach to addressing the complex interplay of obesity, T2DM, and their associated comorbidities.

Acknowledgements

The author acknowledges the use of AI tool for language polishing of the manuscript.

Author details

Fernando Grover Páez*, Sofía Zubieta Barrios, Luz Elena Cortes Bautista, Luis Diego Pantoja Chong and Ximena Guadalupe Reynoso Velazquez
Department of Physiology, Institute of Experimental and Clinical Therapeutics, University Center of Health Sciences, University of Guadalajara, Mexico

*Address all correspondence to: fgroverp@hotmail.com

References

[1] Bray JJH, Foster-Davies H, Salem A, Hoole AL, Obaid DR, Halcox JPJ, et al. Glucagon-like peptide-1 receptor agonists improve biomarkers of inflammation and oxidative stress: A systematic review and meta-analysis of randomised controlled trials. Diabetes, Obesity & Metabolism. 2021;**23**(8):1806-1822. DOI: 10.1111/dom.14399

[2] Frias JP, Nauck MA, Van J, et al. Efficacy and safety of LY3298176, a novel dual GIP and GLP-1 receptor agonist, in patients with type 2 diabetes: A randomized, placebo-controlled and active comparator-controlled phase 2 trial. Lancet. 2018;**392**(10160):2180-2193. DOI: 10.1016/S0140-6736(18)32260-8

[3] Kristensen SL, Rørth R, Jhund PS, et al. Cardiovascular, mortality, and kidney outcomes with GLP-1 receptor agonists in patients with type 2 diabetes: A systematic review and meta-analysis of cardiovascular outcome trials. The Lancet Diabetes and Endocrinology. 2019;7(10):776-785. DOI: 10.1016/S2213-8587(19)30249-9

[4] Finan B, Müller TD, Clemmensen C, Perez-Tilve D, DiMarchi RD, Tschöp MH. Reappraisal of GIP pharmacology for metabolic diseases. Trends in Molecular Medicine. 2016;**22**(5):359-376. DOI: 10.1016/j.molmed.2016.03.005

[5] Wilson JM, Nikooienejad A, Robins DA, et al. The dual glucose-dependent insulinotropic peptide and glucagon-like peptide-1 receptor agonist, tirzepatide, improves lipoprotein biomarkers associated with insulin resistance and cardiovascular risk in patients with type 2 diabetes. Diabetes, Obesity & Metabolism. 2020;**22**(12):2451-2459. DOI: 10.1111/dom.14174

[6] Blüher M, Rosenstock J, Hoefler J, Manuel R, Hennige AM. Dose-response effects on HbA_1c and bodyweight reduction of survodutide, a dual glucagon/GLP-1 receptor agonist, compared with placebo and open-label semaglutide in people with type 2 diabetes: A randomised clinical trial. Diabetologia. 2024;**67**(3):470-482. DOI: 10.1007/s00125-023-06053-9

[7] Lin X, Li H. Obesity: Epidemiology, pathophysiology, and therapeutics. Front Endocrinol (Lausanne). 2021;**12**:706978. DOI: 10.3389/fendo.2021.706978

[8] Busebee B, Ghusn W, Cifuentes L, Acosta A. Obesity: A review of pathophysiology and classification. Mayo Clinic Proceedings. 2023;**98**(12):1842-1857. DOI: 10.1016/j.mayocp.2023.05.026

[9] Wen X, Zhang B, Wu B, Xiao H, Li Z, Li R, et al. Signaling pathways in obesity: Mechanisms and therapeutic interventions. Signal Transduction and Targeted Therapy. 2022;**7**(1):298. DOI: 10.1038/s41392-022-01149-x

[10] Kumar RB, Srivastava G, Reid TJ, Aronne LJ. Understanding the pathophysiologic pathways that underlie obesity and options for treatment. Expert Review of Endocrinology and Metabolism. 2021;**16**(6):321-338. DOI: 10.1080/17446651.2021.1991310

[11] Scheen AJ, Van Gaal LF. Combating the dual burden: Therapeutic targeting of common pathways in obesity and type 2 diabetes. The Lancet Diabetes and Endocrinology. 2014;**2**(11):911-922. DOI: 10.1016/S2213-8587(14)70004-X

[12] Kalra S, Jacob J, Arora S, Kapoor N. The etiopathogenesis and management

of obesity: The quintessential quincunx. The Journal of the Pakistan Medical Association. 2023;**73**(5):1134-1136. DOI: 10.47391/JPMA.23-36

[13] Lastra G, Manrique C, Sowers JR. Obesity and cardiovascular disease: Role of adipose tissue, inflammation, and the renin-angiotensin-aldosterone system. Hormone Molecular Biology and Clinical Investigation. 2013;**15**(2):49-57. DOI: 10.1515/hmbci-2013-0025

[14] Bray GA, Kim KK, JPH W, World Obesity Federation. Obesity: A chronic, relapsing, progressive disease process. Obesity Reviews. 2017;**18**(7):715-723. DOI: 10.1111/obr.12551

[15] Gjermeni E, Kirstein AS, Kolbig F, et al. Obesity- update on the basic pathophysiology and review of recent therapeutic advances. Biomolecules. 2021;**11**(10):1426. DOI: 10.3390/biom11101426

[16] Heymsfield SB, Wadden TA. Mechanisms, pathophysiology, and management of obesity. The New England Journal of Medicine. 2017;**376**(3):254-266. DOI: 10.1056/NEJMra1514009

[17] Zhang Y, Liu J, Yao J, et al. Obesity: Pathophysiology and intervention. Nutrients. 2014;**6**(11):5153-5183. DOI: 10.3390/nu6115153

[18] Pi-Sunyer FX. The medical risks of obesity. Postgraduate Medicine. 2009;**121**(6):21-33. DOI: 10.3810/pgm.2009.11.2074

[19] Kong Y, Yang H, Nie R, et al. Obesity: Pathophysiology and therapeutic interventions. Molecular Biomedicine. 2025;**6**(1):25. DOI: 10.1186/s43556-025-00264-9

[20] Velloso LA, Folli F, Saad MJ. TLR4 at the crossroads of nutrients, gut microbiota, and metabolic inflammation. Endocrine Reviews. 2015;**36**(3):245-271. DOI: 10.1210/er.2014-1100

[21] Tilg H, Moschen AR. Adipocytokines: Mediators linking adipose tissue, inflammation, and immunity. Nature Reviews. Immunology. 2006;**6**(10):772-783. DOI: 10.1038/nri1937

[22] Hotamisligil GS. Inflammation and metabolic disorders. Nature. 2006;**444**(7121):860-867. DOI: 10.1038/nature05485

[23] Donath MY, Shoelson SE. Type 2 diabetes as an inflammatory disease. Nature Reviews. Immunology. 2011;**11**(2):98-107. DOI: 10.1038/nri2925

[24] Szczerbiński L, Florez JC. Precision medicine of obesity as an integral part of type 2 diabetes management—Past, present, and future. The Lancet Diabetes and Endocrinology. 2023;**11**(11):861-878. DOI: 10.1016/S2213-8587(23)00232-2

[25] Drucker DJ. Mechanisms of action and therapeutic application of glucagon-like peptide-1. Cell Metabolism. 2018;**27**(4):740-756. DOI: 10.1016/j.cmet.2018.03.001

[26] Nauck MA, Meier JJ. Incretin hormones: Their role in health and disease. Diabetes, Obesity & Metabolism. 2018;**20**(Suppl 1):5-21. DOI: 10.1111/dom.13129

[27] Holst JJ, Madsbad S. Mechanisms of surgical control of type 2 diabetes: GLP-1 is a key factor. Surgery for Obesity and Related Diseases. 2016;**12**(6):1236-1242. DOI: 10.1016/j.soard.2016.02.033

[28] Jiang Y, Zhu H, Gong F. Why does GLP-1 agonist combined with GIP and/or GCG agonist have greater weight loss effect than GLP-1 agonist alone in obese

adults without type 2 diabetes? Diabetes, Obesity & Metabolism. 2025;**27**(3):1079-1095. DOI: 10.1111/dom.16106

[29] Müller TD, Finan B, Clemmensen C, DiMarchi RD, Tschöp MH. The new biology and pharmacology of glucagon. Physiological Reviews. 2017;**97**(2):721-766. DOI: 10.1152/physrev.00025.2016

[30] Capozzi ME, DiMarchi RD, Tschöp MH, et al. Targeting the incretin/glucagon system with triagonists to treat diabetes. Endocrine Reviews. 2018;**39**(5):719-738. DOI: 10.1210/er.2018-00117

[31] Brandt SJ, Müller TD, DiMarchi RD, Tschöp MH, Stemmer K. Peptide-based multi-agonists: A new paradigm in metabolic pharmacology. Journal of Internal Medicine. 2018;**284**(6):581-602. DOI: 10.1111/joim.12837

[32] Coskun T, Urva S, Roell WC, et al. LY3437943, a novel triple glucagon, GIP, and GLP-1 receptor agonist for glycemic control and weight loss: From discovery to clinical proof of concept. Cell Metabolism. 2022;**34**(9):1234-1247.e9. DOI: 10.1016/j.cmet.2022.07.013

[33] Wharton S, Calanna S, Davies M, et al. Gastrointestinal tolerability of once-weekly semaglutide 2.4 mg in adults with overweight or obesity, and the relationship between gastrointestinal adverse events and weight loss. Diabetes, Obesity & Metabolism. 2022;**24**(1):94-105. DOI: 10.1111/dom.14551

[34] Kaore SBB, Khasbage S, Atal S. Evaluating the efficacy and safety of Tirzepatide on Glycaemic and non-glycaemic outcomes in diabetes: A systematic review of meta-analyses. Cureus. 2024;**16**(3):e56939. DOI: 10.7759/cureus.56939

[35] Min T, Bain SC. The role of tirzepatide, dual GIP and GLP-1 receptor agonist, in the management of type 2 diabetes: The SURPASS clinical trials. Diabetes Therapy. 2021;**12**(1):143-157. DOI: 10.1007/s13300-020-00981-0

[36] Jastreboff AM, Aronne LJ, Ahmad NN, et al. Tirzepatide once weekly for the treatment of obesity. The New England Journal of Medicine. 2022;**387**(3):205-216. DOI: 10.1056/NEJMoa2206038

[37] Wilding JPH, Batterham RL, Calanna S, et al. Once-weekly semaglutide in adults with overweight or obesity. The New England Journal of Medicine. 2021;**384**(11):989-1002. DOI: 10.1056/NEJMoa2032183

[38] Fornes A, Huff J, Pritchard RI. Godfrey M once-weekly semaglutide for weight management: A clinical review. The Journal of Pharmacy Technology. 2022;**38**(4):239-246. DOI: 10.1177/87551225221092681

[39] Wadden TA, Bailey TS, Billings LK, et al. Effect of subcutaneous semaglutide vs placebo as an adjunct to intensive behavioral therapy on body weight in adults with overweight or obesity: The STEP 3 randomized clinical trial. JAMA. 2021;**325**(14):1403-1413. DOI: 10.1001/jama.2021.1831

[40] Garvey WT, Batterham RL, Bhatta M, et al. Two-year effects of semaglutide in adults with overweight or obesity: The STEP 5 trial. Nature Medicine. 2022;**28**(10):2083-2091. DOI: 10.1038/s41591-022-02026-4. epub 2022 Oct 10

[41] Davies M, Færch L, Jeppesen OK, Pakseresht A, et al. Semaglutide 2.4 mg once a week in adults with overweight or obesity, and type 2 diabetes (STEP 2): A randomised, double-blind, double-dummy, placebo-controlled, phase 3 trial. Lancet. 2021;**397**(10278):971-984. DOI: 10.1016/S0140-6736(21)00213-0

[42] Ahrén B, Masmiquel L, Kumar H, et al. Efficacy and safety of once-weekly semaglutide versus once-daily sitagliptin as an add-on to metformin, thiazolidinediones, or both, in patients with type 2 diabetes (SUSTAIN 2): A 56-week, double-blind, phase 3a, randomised trial. The Lancet Diabetes and Endocrinology. 2017;**5**(5):341-354. DOI: 10.1016/S2213-8587(17)30092-X

[43] Marso SP, Daniels GH, Brown-Frandsen K, et al. Liraglutide and cardiovascular outcomes in type 2 diabetes. The New England Journal of Medicine. 2016;**375**(4):311-322. DOI: 10.1056/NEJMoa1603827

[44] Drucker DJ. Mechanisms of action and therapeutic application of glucagon-like Peptide-1. Cell Metabolism. 2018;**27**(4):740-756. DOI: 10.1016/j.cmet.2018.03.001

[45] Nauck MA, Quast DR, Wefers J, Meier JJ. GLP-1 receptor agonists in the treatment of type 2 diabetes—State-of-the-art. Molecular Metabolism. 2021;**46**:101102. DOI: 10.1016/j.molmet.2020.101102

[46] Finan B, Müller TD, Clemmensen C, DiMarchi RD, Tschöp MH. Reappraisal of GIP pharmacology for metabolic diseases. Trends in Molecular Medicine. 2016;**22**(5):359-376. DOI: 10.1016/j.molmed.2016.03.005

[47] Drucker DJ, Habener JF, Holst JJ. Discovery, characterization, and clinical development of the glucagon-like peptides. The Journal of Clinical Investigation. 2017;**127**(12):4217-4227. DOI: 10.1172/JCI97233

[48] Campbell JE, Drucker DJ. Pharmacology, physiology, and mechanisms of incretin hormone action. Cell Metabolism. 2013;**17**(6):819-837. DOI: 10.1016/j.cmet.2013.04.008

[49] Marso SP, Bain SC, Consoli A, et al. Semaglutide and cardiovascular outcomes in patients with type 2 diabetes. The New England Journal of Medicine. 2016;**375**(19):1834-1844. DOI: 10.1056/NEJMoa1607141

[50] Ussher JR, Drucker DJ. Glucagon-like peptide 1 receptor agonists: Cardiovascular benefits and mechanisms of action. Nature Reviews. Cardiology. 2023;**20**(7):463-474. DOI: 10.1038/s41569-023-00849-3

[51] Liu QK. Mechanisms of action and therapeutic applications of GLP-1 and dual GIP/GLP-1 receptor agonists. Frontiers in Endocrinology. 2024;**15**:1431292. DOI: 10.3389/fendo.2024.1431292

[52] Liraglutide and cardiovascular outcomes in type 2 diabetes. The New England Journal of Medicine. 2016;**375**(18):1797. DOI: 10.1056/NEJMc1611289

[53] Wilson JM, Nikooienejad A, Robins DA, Roell WC, et al. The dual glucose-dependent insulinotropic peptide and glucagon-like peptide-1 receptor agonist, tirzepatide, improves lipoprotein biomarkers associated with insulin resistance and cardiovascular risk in patients with type 2 diabetes. Diabetes, Obesity & Metabolism. 2020;**22**(12):2451-2459. DOI: 10.1111/dom.14174

[54] Gallwitz B. Clinical perspectives on the use of the GIP/GLP-1 receptor agonist tirzepatide for the treatment of type-2 diabetes and obesity. Frontiers in Endocrinology. 2022;**13**:1004044. DOI: 10.3389/fendo.2022.1004044

[55] Zheng Z, Zong Y, Ma Y, et al. Glucagon-like peptide-1 receptor: Mechanisms and advances in therapy. Signal Transduction and Targeted

Therapy. 2024;**9**(1):234. DOI: 10.1038/s41392-024-01931-z

[56] Tysoe O. Tirzepatide highly effective for weight loss. Nature Reviews. Endocrinology. 2022;**18**(9):520. DOI: 10.1038/s41574-022-00715-1

[57] Kabahizi A, Wallace B, Lieu L, et al. Glucagon-like peptide-1 (GLP-1) signalling in the brain: From neural circuits and metabolism to therapeutics. British Journal of Pharmacology. 2022;**179**(4):600-624. DOI: 10.1111/bph.15682

[58] Sattar N, Lee MMY, Kristensen SL, et al. Cardiovascular, mortality, and kidney outcomes with GLP-1 receptor agonists in patients with type 2 diabetes: A systematic review and meta-analysis of randomised trials. The Lancet Diabetes and Endocrinology. 2021;**9**(10):653-662. DOI: 10.1016/S2213-8587(21)00203-5

[59] Badve SV, Bilal A, Lee MMY, et al. Effects of GLP-1 receptor agonists on kidney and cardiovascular disease outcomes: A meta-analysis of randomised controlled trials. The Lancet Diabetes and Endocrinology. 2025;**13**(1):15-28. DOI: 10.1016/S2213-8587(24)00271-7

[60] Mahapatra MK, Karuppasamy M, Sahoo BM. Therapeutic potential of semaglutide, a newer GLP-1 receptor agonist, in abating obesity, non-alcoholic steatohepatitis, and neurodegenerative diseases: A narrative review. Pharmaceutical Research. 2022;**39**(6):1233-1248. DOI: 10.1007/s11095-022-03302-1

[61] Siddeeque N, Hussein MH, Abdelmaksoud A, et al. Neuroprotective effects of GLP-1 receptor agonists in neurodegenerative disorders: A large-scale propensity-matched cohort study. International Immunopharmacology. 2024;**143**(Pt 3):113537. DOI: 10.1016/j.intimp.2024.113537

Chapter 5

Lived Experience of Diabetes Self-Management among the Elderly in India

B. Kalpana Kosalram, V. Srinivas and Irene Sambath

Abstract

The World Health Organization (WHO) and the United Nations (UN) designated 2021–2030 as the "Decade of Healthy Ageing," which underscores the increasing importance of addressing the needs of an aging global population. As emphasized in the Longitudinal Aging Study in India (LASI) Wave 1 Report, 2020, India, which is frequently referred to as the "Diabetes Capital of the World," is grappling with a substantial burden of diabetes among older adults. Against this demographic backdrop, the chapter explores the way elderly Indians handle the intricacies of diabetes self-management, which encompasses dietary modifications, medication adherence, physical activity, and routine monitoring, supported by family, healthcare providers, and community resources. This chapter endeavors to inform healthcare professionals, researchers, and policymakers regarding the unique requirements of elderly diabetic patients by providing the reader with personal insights and lived experiences, thereby facilitating a more personalized approach to diabetes care.

Keywords: diabetes self-management, elderly population, older adults, lived experience, aging, India

1. Introduction

The global population is undergoing a significant demographic transition, with an increasing older population. The World Health Organization (WHO) and United Nations (UN) have declared 2021–2030 to be the "Decade of Healthy Ageing" in response to the pressing demands of addressing the health emergencies facing the elderly [1]. In India, the elderly population is increasing at an alarming rate and is approaching crisis levels. The India Aging Report 2023, released by the United Nations Population Fund (UNFPA) and the International Institute for Population Sciences (IIPS), indicates that senior citizens currently make up 10% of India's total population, which is expected to rise to 14.9% by 2036 [2].

Simultaneously, a notable epidemiological transition has been occurring toward chronic diseases, particularly Type 2 Diabetes Mellitus (T2DM). This condition is characterized by inadequate insulin production or reduced insulin sensitivity. Estimates suggest that the population of adults aged 20–79 living with diabetes will rise from 537 million in 2021 to 643 million by 2030, and subsequently to 783 million by 2045 [3]. Diabetes is recognized as a significant public health concern on a global scale. Almost half of these adults are not receiving treatment and are unaware of their condition. The prevalence of diabetes is significantly elevated as individuals age, which is a cause for concern. In 2019, 19.3% of individuals aged 65–99 were diagnosed with diabetes, as per the International Diabetes Federation (IDF). This figure is expected to increase to 195.2 million by 2030 and 276.2 million by 2045 [3].

India, often called the "Diabetes Capital of the World," is home to the largest populace of diabetics. A study by the Noncommunicable Diseases Risk Factor Collaboration (NCD-RisC) and the World Health Organization (WHO) in 2022 shows that India has the most untreated diabetes cases in the world [4]. The International Diabetes Federation estimated 74.7 million people in India aged 20 to 79 lived with diabetes in 2021; this number is expected to increase to 124.9 million by 2045 [3]. The prevalence of diabetes in India has historically varied from 13% to 25%, with higher rates in urban areas and demographically advancing states [5].

The Longitudinal Aging Study in India (LASI) is the first full-scale national survey of scientific investigation of the health, economic, social determinants, and consequences of population aging in India. According to the LASI Wave 1 report, the self-reported prevalence of diabetes mellitus in older adults aged 45–59 and elderly aged 60 and above was 9 and 14%, respectively [6]. Urbanization, diet changes, and the increased incidence of obesity lead to rising numbers of new diabetes cases. At the same time, older people are confronted with atypical presentations of diabetes, comorbidities, and a higher risk of macro- and microvascular complications, leading to increased mortality, functional status decrements, and institutionalization [7].

The diabetes management paradigms comprise several components, with self-management being one of the most significant in the theory and practice of diabetes care. Self-management ranges from adherence to medication to diet and physical activity changes to routine health monitoring. Unfortunately, elderly populations encounter numerous hurdles to effective self-management. The key hurdles include poor-quality health services, inadequate age-targeted counseling, and limited access to age-friendly healthcare technologies. Language barriers, poor communication, visual impairment, cognitive decline, insufficient financial resources, and a dearth of guidelines designed to meet the dietary and physical activity needs of the geriatric population also compound matters. Inequitable healthcare access, especially in secondary and tertiary care, further burdens diabetes complications. Social determinants, including family support, healthcare accessibility, and cultural perceptions of aging and illness, play pivotal roles in shaping their self-management behaviors.

1.1 Qualitative approach and rationale

There is a deepening crisis of diabetes among India's aging population that calls for a deeper understanding of how elderly individuals navigate the complexities of diabetes self-management. As reported in the LASI Wave 1 report, Tamil Nadu ranks third among the Indian states with 10.4% of its people aged 60 and above, following Kerala (12.6%) and Goa (11.2%) [6].

This chapter presents the personal narratives of 10 elderly individuals diagnosed with T2DM, comprising six outpatients and four residents from assisted living facility at a well-known geriatric hospital in Chennai, Tamil Nadu. Their experiences highlight the intricate relationship between personal, social, and systemic factors that affect how they manage their diabetes. Verbatim quotes reveal their challenges, resilience, and coping strategies, providing a deeper insight and nuanced understanding of their everyday realities.

1.2 Basic demographics

Of the ten individuals, six were male, and four were female, aged 69–82 years. All of them had diagnosed T2DM, with 4 and 46 years of disease duration. Four individuals were illiterate, three had primary school education, and three were graduates. All of them were married, two separated from spouse and two widowed. Five individuals had a family history of diabetes. Eight individuals were unemployed, and two were supporting family business. Only one of them availed health insurance supported by the children. Regarding diabetes-related complications, two had diabetic neuropathy, three had cardiovascular symptoms, and two had a diabetic foot. Seven of them had other comorbidities.

2. Challenges in diabetes self-management

Factors such as the physical, psychological, and social challenges experienced by elderly persons with T2DM contribute to the effectiveness of diabetes self-management. These obstacles aggravate their sufferings and the risk of complications and diminishes the overall quality of life.

2.1 Physical limitations and comorbidities

The aging process is generally associated with physical frailty, reduced stamina, and a higher prevalence of comorbidities, which makes diabetes management increasingly challenging. Comorbid conditions like arthritis, obesity, and cardiovascular issues often coexist with diabetes, causing older persons to struggle with their day-to-day activities [7]. These challenges are echoed by one individual who shared, "*I have arthritis which limits my walking. Added to this, my weight issue puts a strain on my knees*" (P1).

Physical impairments also lead to dependence on others, sometimes fostering feelings of being a burden. For instance, another individual mentioned, "*I'm scared to cut my own nails, thinking I might hurt myself. I rely on my grandchildren for such tasks*" (P3). The fear of injuries and delayed wound healing is a constant concern among diabetic elderly individuals, further complicating self-care routines. This aligns with studies that highlight delayed healing is caused by compromised immune responses and vascular complications, which are often accompanied by other chronic conditions like hypertension and dyslipidemia [8]. As one individual noted, "*I have cholesterol and hypertension ... I cannot bend down to lift anything, my head spins. So, I call for help ...*" (P9). Research supports this, indicating that multimorbidity significantly impairs diabetes management in older adults, as they juggle complex medication regimens and lifestyle adjustments [5].

Acceptance of the disease is often a gradual process that emerges through personal reflection and lived experiences. One individual described the journey as a "*...battle with my inner self and the system. I regret not being careful earlier*" (P2). While initial resistance to the diagnosis is common, eventual acceptance enables better disease management. Literature also underscores that acceptance and resilience improve self-care behaviors and emotional well-being among elderly diabetics [9].

Obesity and mental toll were another concern expressed: "*I've never been fat, but now I am. It's really depressing*" (P2). Studies show that obesity not only exacerbates diabetes symptoms but also negatively affects self-image, further complicating self-care efforts [10].

2.2 Psychological and emotional challenges

The burden of living with diabetes comes with a psychological cost, such as stigma, feelings of frustration, and emotional exhaustion. A good number of older people struggle to comprehend the lifelong nature of the disease, intensifying the feelings of helplessness. One individual remarked, "*Diabetes is an exhausting disease that cannot be completely eradicated; it is both physically and mentally painful*" (P5).

The stigma associated with the condition can also be socially isolating. For example, a participant shared, "*I'm tired of being called a diabetic... It's a label I will carry for the rest of my life*" (P4). Stigmatization is common, with studies noting that it often discourages individuals from openly discussing their condition, hindering access to support systems.

Coping strategies such as concealing one's condition are often employed. For instance, a participant recalled, "*I preferred to keep my condition discreet, but my unexplained weight loss was spotted by my colleagues. The news spread...*" (P3). Though such strategies may offer temporary relief that is situation and context specific to the individual, it can lead to feelings of loneliness and decreased emotional well-being.

The concept of the "diminished self" emerged from participants' narratives, where they compared their current state to their past healthier selves. One participant reflected, "*I regret not having looked after myself in the past, but now I have come to terms with it*" (P8). This aligns with studies suggesting that individuals often go through a transformation, a phase of psychological distress, marked by a shift from self-blame to acceptance and adaptation [11].

The intersection of physical health and emotions can take a toll on mental health, as expressed by a participant: "*I went from being confident to somebody drained and angry*" (P4). Emotional distress, coupled with diabetes, can lead to poor glycaemic control and further complications, underscoring the importance of psychological interventions in diabetes care [11].

2.3 Social and environmental barriers

Environmental factors play a significant role in shaping diabetes self-management. Participants frequently reported feeling stigmatized ("diabetes stigma" [12] or unsupported in social settings. For instance, one individual shared, "*I avoid weddings and family gatherings due to my frailty. I also fear being questioned*" (P10). This aligns with studies indicating that societal stigma can lead to social withdrawal, reducing access to support networks [12].

Environmental challenges, such as inadequate disabled-friendly facilities, further limit mobility and independence. One participant recalled, "*I once dined out and felt giddy but couldn't find a rail to hold onto*" (P5). Another shared, "*I prefer a wheelchair, but not many places have ramps*" (P7). Research corroborates these experiences, emphasizing that infrastructural barriers significantly impact the quality of life for elderly individuals with diabetes [13].

Finally, the economic burden of diabetes also emerged as a barrier. The cost of medications, frequent health checkups, and lifestyle modifications often strained financial resources, further complicating disease management. This challenge is well-documented in literature, where the financial strain of managing chronic illnesses disproportionately affects elderly individuals on fixed incomes [13].

3. Strategies for self-management

Managing Type 2 Diabetes Mellitus (T2DM) among elderly individuals is multi-faceted, involving physical, psychological, and social dimensions.

3.1 Dietary adjustments and food-related practices

Dietary management emerged as a critical yet challenging aspect of diabetes self-care, which is heavily influenced by socioeconomic factors, cultural beliefs, and limited nutritional education. Cultural norms around food preparation and meal composition may clash with clinical dietary recommendations, as medical advice is not always tailored to individuals' socio-cultural realities, particularly for those relying on traditional diets or experiencing food insecurity [13, 14].

Limited nutritional education often results in simplistic views about diabetes management, such as focusing solely on reducing sugar intake. For example, one participant shared, "*Diet is not just about avoiding sweets; it also involves eating smaller, more frequent meals*" (P2), while another said, "*I rely on supplies from the ration shop. I don't get to eat much vegetables. It's mostly lentils and rice*" (P5). The decline in traditional, nutrient-rich foods and the adoption of processed, energy-dense diets reflect a shift in dietary habits contributing to poor diabetes control as explained by one individual "*My children sometimes order biryani and desserts from food delivery app. When there is no home cooked food, I eat this ordered food which is too salty and heavy to digest*" (P1).

Financial constraints compounded dietary challenges, with participants often unable to afford balanced meals. Many rely on low-cost, calorie-dense foods, which do not meet nutritional needs, contributing to poor diabetes control. One individual remarked, "*I cannot afford healthy groceries by myself. If my son's family willingly share chicken or fish, I eat. Otherwise, it's only during festive occasions*" (P10).

3.2 Medication adherence

It was interesting to observe varied attitudes toward medication adherence that were primarily influenced by the individual's beliefs. Mistrust in allopathic medicine also surfaced from the verbatims. Participants sometimes turned to alternative therapies based on cultural beliefs or anecdotal advice. This is a typical treatment-seeking behavior of persons especially from rural India. For example, one participant stated, "*I switched to traditional medicine but didn't experience benefits, so I resumed allopathic treatment*" (P10). Additionally, the "pill burden" from managing multiple comorbidities discouraged adherence: "*I have a pile of medicines to take every day. I wonder whether my body can cope*" (P2).

3.3 Incorporation of physical activity

The trinity of barriers—personal (e.g., frailty, lack of motivation), societal (e.g., lack of support), and environmental (e.g., unsafe surroundings)—restricted participants' ability to incorporate physical activity into their routines [15]. For example, one individual said, "*I don't have space inside my house to walk. The house is on a busy street, so I sit or lie down most of the time*" (P3). Unsafe surroundings, lack of open spaces, and unsuitable infrastructure discourage elderly individuals from regular outdoor physical activities. These challenges are particularly acute in urban environments, where busy streets or overcrowded living conditions restrict safe and comfortable spaces for walking or exercise.

Senior persons with higher BMI are more likely to avoid physical activity, with diseases such as arthritis or cardiovascular conditions further limiting participation. "*I have a big belly and breathing difficulties. I cannot do much…*" (P7). Fatigue, lacking companionship during walking, and low motivation were also identified as significant challenges for this demographic.

Despite this, some participants creatively integrated light activities like cleaning or gardening into their daily lives. For example, one participant noted, "*I do some gardening in the evenings but don't walk intentionally due to my frailty*" (P1). These activities help improve mobility and well-being without requiring strenuous effort or specialized facilities.

3.4 Self-monitoring practices and tools

Self-monitoring of blood glucose was inconsistently practiced among participants. While some used glucometers regularly, others relied on subjective feelings to assess their glucose levels. One participant admitted, "*I haven't measured it for a long time; sometimes, when I feel my blood sugar rising, I take a measurement*" (P4). The cost of glucometers and strips was a limiting factor for some, with several relying on donated equipment.

While some recognized its importance, others struggled with consistency due to the invasive nature of glucose monitoring, side effects, or fear of dependency. One participant shared, "*In the beginning, I was consistent in checking my blood glucose. But I found it troublesome and stopped measuring frequently*" (P9). Others expressed apprehension about the pain involved in blood sugar checks "*I don't want to measure my blood sugar because it hurts my fingers*" (P3). Research indicates that invasive glucose monitoring methods creates anxiety and fear. Many patients discontinue frequent checks or reluctant to practice home testing due to the discomfort caused by finger-prick tests [16].

4. Role of support systems

Effective diabetes self-management extends beyond individual effort, relying on robust support systems: family and caregivers, healthcare providers, and community resources.

4.1 Family and caregiver involvement

Family dynamics play a significant role in the self-management of diabetes among elderly individuals. The shift in family roles, as seen in multigenerational households, often affects dietary habits and time for exercise. For instance, one individual shared, "*I live with my son's family. I have three grandchildren to take care. It is difficult to find free time to exercise*" (P5).

In cases where elderly individuals lacked immediate family support, their emotional well-being was often compromised. As one participant recounted, "*I was living with the support of my cousins after my family members passed away. The neighbours and others looked down on me for being a burden to them. I felt helpless and hopeless*" (P8).

4.2 Healthcare provider support

The elderly individuals highlighted challenges in accessing and utilizing healthcare services, particularly due to aging-related factors like memory decline and sensory impairments. For example, one participant stated, "*I try to remember what my doctor says, but I tend to forget about it*" (P6). Others, like P8, emphasized difficulties in understanding written health information due to vision problems.

Negative experiences in public healthcare facilities, such as unapproachable staff and long wait times, were demotivating. "*Sometimes I want to ask the doctor, but they are busy and unavailable*" (P4). Individuals often valued private healthcare more for its perceived better communication and attentiveness. One of them observed, "*To be honest…counselling us needs a kind approach. Comforting and soothing words help with our distress. Being stern will stop us from asking doubts*" (P1).

Social interactions and conversational support emerged as a crucial coping mechanism. Individuals emphasized the importance of talking to healthcare professionals, peers, or friends. One remarked, "*The less you choose to talk to your doctor about your health problem, the slower your recovery…*" (P9). Studies confirm that open communication fosters emotional resilience and provides practical guidance for managing diabetes [13].

4.3 Community resources and peer support

Community and peer networks emerged as invaluable resources for participants. In assisted living facilities, peers often became substitutes for distant or uninvolved family members. "In this assisted living, my children from US send money every month but don't check on me often. It is the doctors and fellow inmates who I rely on for moral support" (P9). Peer interactions provided emotional support and a platform to share experiences, fostering a sense of understanding and solidarity.

Accessibility to healthcare services was another challenge, especially in rural areas. One participant described the logistical hurdles: "*When I was initially diagnosed, I was residing in my village. Getting to the health centre was a nightmare due to limited daily bus schedules and poor roads*" (P7). Spiritual practices and community gatherings, such as attending temples or listening to bhajans, were highlighted as stress-relieving and therapeutic. "*I forget my stress when I listen to bhajans… it is mind-relaxing*" (P5).

Individuals also highlighted the value of shared experiences in fostering self-awareness and motivation. One participant shared, "*Whenever I meet others in the OPD like me, I believe time has been the best healer*" (P9), underscoring the psychological benefits of peer support.

5. Cultural and socioeconomic influences

Cultural perceptions of aging and illness, along with financial challenges, deeply impacts the management of T2DM.

5.1 Cultural perceptions of aging and illness

Cultural attitudes toward aging and illness influence how individuals perceive and manage this chronic condition. Some expressed indifference perceiving their condition as an inevitable consequence of aging or beyond their control, as exemplified by one individual who stated, "*I just let it be. I'm tired of thinking about my condition*" (P6). Another participant admitted to requiring external reminders due to their lack of concern "*I need reminders as I fail to care about my disease*" (P7).

This detachment from self-care was often linked to a perceived lack of symptoms or the belief that diabetes was not a serious condition unless complications arose, attributing it to external factors such as diet or fate. For instance, one participant reflected, "*I used to eat whatever grew in my farm. I didn't expect to fall sick, and I didn't really pay much attention to it because there weren't any symptoms*" (P4).

Religious and spiritual beliefs also played a significant role in shaping health behaviors. Another individual associated diabetes with divine punishment or spiritual trial, stating, "*Initially, I thought it was a curse from God and met my community's faith leader for a remedy. I was given traditional medicines*" (P10).

5.2 Economic constraints and access to healthcare

Economic hardships were pervasive among participants, significantly affecting their ability to manage diabetes. High healthcare costs, including those for diagnostic tests and medications, often led to compromised care. One individual expressed frustration: "*Doctors ask for fasting sugar tests. I cannot afford private labs all the time. If I opt for the public health facility, it is crowded and adds to the difficulty of waiting without food*" (P6).

Another described turning to government-subsidized options due to rising cost of living and inadequate financial support: "*My pension has stopped. Everything has become expensive now. Purchasing medicines from private pharmacies is beyond my capacity, so I buy from Jan Aushadhi stores*" (P4).

Not possessing health insurance is a burden on the out-of-pocket medical expenses, often at the expense of other necessities. Many believed from personal experiences or from peer reference that private healthcare facilities offer superior services, which led them to prioritize quality over affordability despite financial strain. This often forced them to make difficult choices, such as deciding which medications to purchase. As one participant lamented, "*Out-of-pocket expenses often make me skip some medicines my doctor prescribes*" (P5).

6. Implications for practice

6.1 Recommendations for healthcare providers

It goes without saying that the healthcare providers from both private and government settings collaborate with multidisciplinary teams to deliver holistic care and assistance to elderly diabetic patients amidst the structural and systemic challenges. Considering the unique challenges faced by elderly individuals managing T2DM due to physical frailty, comorbid conditions, and mobility challenges, healthcare providers must adopt a comprehensive approach that integrates medical, psychological, and social interventions. Given the complexities of managing diabetes alongside other chronic conditions, simplify the self-care regimens by integrating strategies for managing multiple conditions into a unified diabetic care plan. Assistive devices could be recommended for individuals with physical limitations. Implementing domiciliary visits by healthcare workers to bridge access gaps, especially for immobile or dependent patients.

Family-centered care enhances glycaemic control and improves treatment adherence. Healthcare providers must educate patients and families on affordable and locally available nutritious food options, about the risks of delayed wound healing, provide specific wound care guidance to mitigate complications, emphasize the importance of using affordable and user-friendly glucose monitoring device, clearly explaining the progressive nature of diabetes through simplified health education materials, and the role of medications in preventing complications. Healthcare providers should recommend practical and accessible forms of exercise such as low-impact activities like chair yoga, stretches, or short neighborhood walks and advocate for community-based initiatives that reduce environmental barriers to diabetes management, such as unsafe exercise spaces or inaccessible healthcare facilities. For elderly patients facing economic constraints, guidance must be provided regarding affordable resources such as government-supported stores for generic medicines, and visiting nearest primary health center or hospital.

The psychological burden of diabetes, including feelings of stigma, frustration, and emotional exhaustion, necessitates mental health support. The patient-provider relationship is a cornerstone of alleviating their fear, building trust, and supporting consistent habits of diabetes management. Encouraging open conversations about the challenges of living with diabetes and normalizing discussions about stigma can encourage patients to access support networks and counseling services without fear of judgment. Open communication through empathetic, culturally sensitive dialog in the form of workshops or group sessions fosters emotional resilience, creates safe spaces where elderly diabetics can share experiences and strategies, and helps elderly patients navigate their self-care routines. This extends to conversational and emotional support from peers. Healthcare facilities may provide family education about the chronic nature of diabetes, to reduce self-blame, promote understanding, and assist in routine diabetes management tasks.

6.2 Policy considerations and initiatives for diabetes elderly are

The increasing prevalence of diabetes among India's elderly population necessitates large-scale implementation of periodic diabetes screening programs targeting adults aged 45 and above to facilitate early detection and timely intervention, and comprehensive public health campaigns to raise awareness about the disease. Ayushman Bharat Health and Wellness Centres already play a critical role in this area by offering screenings for common NCDs, including diabetes [17]. Initiatives like the Fit India Movement and yoga programs by the Ministry of AYUSH have tailored programs to include physical activity regimens for the elderly [17, 18]. Collaboration with organizations like the Food Safety and Standards Authority of India (FSSAI) can encourage the adoption of balanced diets to prevent and manage diabetes [17].

Healthcare access and affordability remain critical challenges for older adults, particularly in rural areas. Under the National Programme for Prevention and Control of Cancer, Diabetes, Cardiovascular Diseases, and Stroke (NPCDCS) which was renamed the National Programme for Prevention & Control of Non-Communicable Diseases (NP-NCD) in May 2023, financial assistance is offered for purchasing glucometers and diabetes medications, as requested by states and Union Territories [17]. The National Health Mission's (NHM) Free Drugs Service Initiative provides free essential medications, including insulin to economically vulnerable groups [17]. Generic medications including insulin at affordable prices are available at The Pradhan Mantri Bhartiya Janaushadhi Pariyojana (PMBJP) [17]. A dedicated "Vay Vandana Card" under the Ayushman Bharat Pradhan Mantri Jan Arogya Yojana (AB PM-JAY) provides free annual health coverage of up to Rs 5 lakh to eligible senior citizens aged 70 and above [19].

Doorstep healthcare delivery programs like Tamil Nadu's 'Makkalai Thedi Maruthuvam' (a comprehensive set of 'home-based health care services' to ensure a continuum of care and meet the health needs of beneficiaries in the family) should be scaled nationally to ensure equitable access to essential medicines and regular follow-up care for elderly patients, particularly in underserved areas [20]. The recent initiative by the Directorate of Public Health and Preventive Medicine, The Government of Tamil Nadu by introducing simplified flowcharts through the implementation of the 'Comprehensive Step-wise Approach for Hypertension and Diabetes Management' has exemplified the importance of standardized protocols at the primary care level [21]. Guiding the patients and their families to these government-led initiatives must be prioritized to help elderly diabetic persons significantly reduce out-of-pocket expenditure.

Targeted policy measures can address health system inequities. Precision public health approaches, such as decentralized care cascade models, can track the progression of diabetes from diagnosis to management across states, addressing regional disparities. Strengthening primary healthcare centers and training healthcare workers to provide age-sensitive diabetes care is essential. Public health expenditure in India continues to remain low compared to the international level of health spending. Increased budget allocations for diabetes care, particularly for preventive and management services, are crucial to reduce economic inequalities.

In a country with substantial diabetes burden, it is surprising that India's contribution toward global diabetes research is disproportionately low. However, a predominant initiative by India is the Longitudinal Aging Study in India (LASI), which is envisioned to be conducted every 5 years for the next 25 years, with Wave 1 survey conducted in 2017–2018 and Wave 2 survey in 2024–2025 [6]. It is well-positioned to evaluate the effect of changing policies on the behavioral outcomes in India providing a vital database for designing age-specific diabetes interventions. Initiatives like the Simple App under the India Hypertension Control Initiative (IHCI) demonstrate the potential of user-centered, point-of-care applications in improving diabetes management [22]. Scaling such technologies can enhance monitoring and care delivery in busy public health facilities.

Further, randomized controlled trials and multicomponent interventions tailored for aging populations are critical for evidence-based policy formulation. In diabetic patients, psychological distress, also known as diabetes-related distress (DRD), is under-recognized and undertreated emphasizing the critical need for drug discovery [11]. New innovations in non-injectable insulin options such as transdermal patches and inhalable insulin, also studying their long-term efficacy, safety, and cost-effectiveness, will be a significant step forward in addressing barriers posed by needle-phobia in diabetes management. Precision medicine research, leveraging big data analytics, can help tailor personalized drug treatment plans and lifestyle interventions. Future research should address the social determinants of health affecting diabetes-related outcomes [15]. Adopting multidisciplinary frameworks and methodologies in future research approaches supported by funding bodies can fill knowledge gaps and offer evidenced data regarding global and regional variations to address disparities in diabetes health outcomes. At the global level, an international consensus statement and a unanimous pledge was published in 2024 to accelerate an end to diabetes stigma and discrimination [23].

7. Conclusions

Not only social and environmental factors but also the individual's own complex perceptions and experiences shape their management of Type 2 Diabetes Mellitus (T2DM) in the elderly population in India. Though self-management is a cornerstone of diabetes care, the personal narratives highlight that it is fraught with challenges such as psychological burdens, physical frailty, and limited social and environmental support. Financial hardships, cultural perceptions, and the stigma associated with diabetes further complicate the journey of managing this chronic lifelong condition. Despite these hurdles, many individuals demonstrated resilience by adopting creative coping strategies, including light physical activities, dietary adjustments, and seeking support from peers and caregivers.

Their findings reinforce the urgent need for holistic and inclusive diabetes care tailored to the unique needs of the elderly in India. Healthcare providers must integrate medical, psychological, and social interventions with the personalized patient-centered approach. Policymakers should prioritize in their planning and implementation: affordable healthcare access, community-based resources, and culturally sensitive health education. Bridging these gaps can empower elderly diabetics to achieve better health outcomes and improve their quality of life.

Acknowledgements

We sincerely thank Geri Care Hospital for facilitating patient interactions, which greatly contributed to the depth and relevance of this study.

Conflict of interest

The authors declare no conflict of interest.

Thanks

We are deeply grateful to the patients who generously shared their time and experiences, providing invaluable insights that were central to this study.

Acronyms and abbreviations

AB PM-JAY	Ayushman Bharat Pradhan Mantri Jan Arogya Yojana
AYUSH	Ayurveda, Yoga, and Naturopathy, Unani, Siddha, and Homeopathy
DRD	diabetes-related distress
FSSAI	Food Safety and Standards Authority of India

IHCI	India Hypertension Control Initiative
IIPS	International Institute for Population Sciences
LASI	Longitudinal Aging Study in India
NPCDCS	National Programme for Prevention and Control of Cancer, Diabetes, Cardiovascular Diseases, and Stroke
NCD-RisC	Non-communicable Diseases Risk Factor Collaboration
NHM	National Health Mission
NP-NCD	National Programme for Prevention & Control of Non-Communicable Diseases
PMBJP	Pradhan Mantri Bhartiya Janaushadhi Pariyojana
T2DM	Type 2 Diabetes Mellitus
UN	United Nations
UNFPA	United Nations Population Fund

Author details

B. Kalpana Kosalram[1*], V. Srinivas[2] and Irene Sambath[1]

1 SRM School of Public Health, SRM Institute of Science and Technology, Kattankulathur, Chengalpattu, India

2 Geri Care Hospital, Chennai, Tamil Nadu

*Address all correspondence to: kalpax4@gmail.com

References

[1] World Health Organization. UN Decade of Healthy Ageing: Plan of Action 2021-2030 [Internet]. 2020. Available from: https://www.who.int/initiatives/decade-of-healthy-ageing

[2] International Institute for Population Sciences & United Nations Population Fund 2023. India Ageing Report 2023, Caring for our Elders: Institutional Responses. New Delhi: United Nations Population Fund. p. 2020

[3] IDF Diabetes Atlas [Internet]. 10th ed. Brussels, Belgium: International Diabetes Federation; 2021. Available from: https://www.diabetesatlas.org

[4] Zhou B, Rayner AW, Gregg EW, Sheffer KE, Carrillo-Larco RM, Bennett JE, et al. Worldwide trends in diabetes prevalence and treatment from 1990 to 2022: A pooled analysis of 1108 population-representative studies with 141 million participants. Lancet. 2024;**404**(10467):2077-2093. DOI: 10.1016/S0140-6736(24)02317-1

[5] Maiti S, Akhtar S, Upadhyay AK, Mohanty SK. Socioeconomic inequality in awareness, treatment and control of diabetes among adults in India: Evidence from National Family Health Survey of India (NFHS), 2019-2021. Scientific Reports. 2023;**13**(1):2971. DOI: 10.1038/s41598-023-29978-y

[6] International Institute for Population Sciences (IIPS), National Programme for Health Care of Elderly (NPHCE), MoHFW HTHCS of PH (HSPH), The U of SC (USC). Longitudinal Ageing Study in India (LASI) Wave 1, 2017-18, India Report. Mumbai: International Institute for Population Sciences; 2020

[7] Sinclair A, Saeedi P, Kaundal A, Karuranga S, Malanda B, Williams R. Diabetes and global ageing among 65-99-year-old adults: Findings from the International Diabetes Federation Diabetes Atlas, 9th edition. Diabetes Research and Clinical Practice. Apr 2020;**162**:108078. DOI: 10.1016/j.diabres.2020.108078

[8] Guan H, Tian J, Wang Y, Niu P, Zhang Y, Zhang Y, et al. Advances in secondary prevention mechanisms of macrovascular complications in type 2 diabetes mellitus patients: A comprehensive review. European Journal of Medical Research. 2024;**29**(1):152. DOI: 10.1186/s40001-024-01739-1

[9] Kusnanto K, Arifin H, Widyawati IY. A qualitative study exploring diabetes resilience among adults with regulated type 2 diabetes mellitus. Diabetes & Metabolic Syndrome: Clinical Research. 2020;**14**(6):1681-1687. Available from: https://www.sciencedirect.com/science/article/pii/S1871402120303386

[10] American Diabetes Association Professional Practice Committee. Obesity and weight management for the prevention and treatment of type 2 diabetes: Standards of care in diabetes–2024. Diabetes Care. 1 Jan 2023;**47**(Suppl. 1):S145-S157. DOI: 10.2337/dc24-S008

[11] Akshatha S, Nayak UB. The psychological distress associated with type 2 diabetes mellitus represents an unmet need for drug discovery. Medicine in Drug Discovery. 2024;**23**:100196. Available from: https://www.sciencedirect.com/science/article/pii/S2590098624000216

[12] Sri A, Lakshmi G, Srid G. Stigma in Type 2 diabetes: A study from Southern

India. Discover Mental Health; 2024. DOI: 10.21203/rs.3.rs-5354625/v1

[13] Wangnoo SK, Maji D, Das AK, Rao PV, Moses A, Sethi B, et al. Barriers and solutions to diabetes management: An Indian perspective. Indian Journal of Endocrinology and Metabolism. 2013;**17**(4):594-601

[14] Viswanathan V, Krishnan D, Kalra S, Chawla R, Tiwaskar M, Saboo B, et al. Insights on medical nutrition therapy for type 2 diabetes mellitus: An Indian perspective. Advances in Therapy. 2019;**36**(3):520-547. DOI: 10.1007/s12325-019-0872-8

[15] Hill-Briggs F, Adler NE, Berkowitz SA, Chin MH, Gary-Webb TL, Navas-Acien A, et al. Social determinants of health and diabetes: A scientific review. Diabetes Care. 2020;**44**(1):258-279. DOI: 10.2337/dci20-0053

[16] Pamungkas RA, Chamroonsawasdi K. Psychological problems related to capillary blood glucose testing and insulin injection among diabetes patients. Frontiers of Nursing. 2020;7(2):87-95. DOI: 10.2478/fon-2020-0015

[17] Ministry of Health and Family Welfare India. World Diabetes Day 2024. India: Press Information Bureau; 2024. Available from: https://mohfw.gov.in/?q=/press-info/7883

[18] Ministry of Youth Affairs & Sports, The Government of India. Fitness Protocols and Guidelines for 65+ Years. India: Fit India Mission; 2020. Available from: http://fitindia.gov.in/

[19] Ministry of Health and Family Welfare India. Ayushman Vay Vandana Cards. India: Press Information Bureau; 2024. Available from: https://pib.gov.in/PressReleasePage.aspx?PRID=2082288

[20] State Planning Commission. Makkalai Thedi Maruthuvam (Medicine in Search of People). Tamil Nadu, India: The Government of Tamil Nadu; 2023. Available from: https://spc.tn.gov.in/ta/makkalai-thedi-maruthuvam-tamil/

[21] The Hindu. Public Health Directorate Issues Protocols for Hypertension, Diabetes Management At Primary Care Level2024. pp. 1-2. Available from: https://www.thehindu.com/news/cities/chennai/public-health-directorate-issues-protocols-for-hypertension-diabetes-management-at-primary-care-level/article68973162.ece

[22] Ganeshkumar P, Bhatnagar A, Burka D, Durgad K, Krishna A, Das B, et al. Discovery, development, and deployment of a user-centered point-of-care digital information system to treat and track hypertension and diabetes patients under India Hypertension Control Initiative 2019-2022, India. Digit Health. 2024;**1**(10):20552076241250150. DOI: 10.1177/20552076241250153

[23] Speight J, Holmes-Truscott E, Garza M, Scibilia R, Wagner S, Kato A, et al. Bringing an end to diabetes stigma and discrimination: An international consensus statement on evidence and recommendations. The Lancet Diabetes and Endocrinology. 2024;**12**(1):61-82

Chapter 6

Sarcopenia and Type 2 Diabetes Mellitus: Evaluation, Pathophysiological Links, and Management Strategies

Jaya Bhanu Kanwar

Abstract

Sarcopenia refers to the rapid loss of skeletal muscle mass and strength, which can result in serious consequences such as falls, fractures, and a higher risk of mortality. The prevalence of sarcopenia is observed to be twice as high in individuals with type 2 diabetes mellitus. Notably, there is a bidirectional relationship between sarcopenia and type 2 diabetes mellitus, where each condit--ion can exacerbate the progression of the other. Overlapping pathophysiological mechanisms, such as insulin resistance, inflammation, oxidative stress, accumulation of advanced glycation end products, mitochondrial dysfunction, myosteatosis, and the aging process itself contribute to the development of both conditions. A few treatments, such as myostatin antagonists, testosterone supplementation, and selective androgen receptor modulators have been explored, but many remain in the experimental or clinical trial stages. The cornerstone of management involves nutritional intervention with foods rich in protein, essential amino acids, vitamin D, and omega-3 fatty acids. Additionally, incorporating regular physical activity, particularly resistance exercises, and minimizing sedentary behavior are key components for management of sarcopenia.

Keywords: sarcopenia, type 2 diabetes mellitus, pathophysiological links, myosteatosis, nutritional intervention

1. Introduction

Sarcopenia is defined by a rapid decline in skeletal muscle mass and strength. When this decline occurs primarily as a result of aging, it is referred to as primary sarcopenia. In contrast, when it is caused by underlying conditions such as malignancy, chronic renal failure, HIV infection, cardiovascular disease, or liver disorders; it is termed secondary sarcopenia [1]. The rate of muscle mass decline is estimated to be around 8% per decade up to the age of 70. After this point, the rate of loss accelerates to approximately 13–24% per decade [2]. This decline in muscle mass leads to poor physical performance as well as have adverse effects like fall, fractures, and increased mortality [3, 4]. Sarcopenia was officially recognized as a distinct disease

 IntechOpen

entity in 2016 and was assigned a code in International Classification of Diseases-10 clinical modification (ICD10-CM) [5]. Skeletal muscle plays a crucial role in type 2 diabetes mellitus (T2DM) as it is one of the primary tissues responsible for glucose utilization and the largest insulin-sensitive tissue in the body. This makes it essential for maintaining energy balance and metabolic homeostasis [6]. People with T2DM are at high risk for developing sarcopenia as compared to normal population [7]. There exists a bidirectional relationship between sarcopenia and T2DM, with each condition influencing the progression of the other. Additionally, sarcopenia is now being recognized as a long-term complication of T2DM, similar to other long-term complications.

2. Epidemiology

The age-related sarcopenia is estimated to affect 5–10% of the general population [1], while 10–27% of older adults have sarcopenia [8]. A recent cross-sectional study involving 6381 adults over the age of 50, using data retrieved from the National Health and Nutrition Examination Survey, found that the prevalence of sarcopenia was 28% among individuals with T2DM compared to 16% in those without T2DM [9]. A longitudinal study conducted among elderly community dwellers (aged over 60 years) included 27,241 participants and found that sarcopenia was prevalent in 27.0% of them. Participants with diabetes had a significantly higher odds ratio of 1.14 for developing sarcopenia [10]. A study involving 824 older Japanese adults found that individuals with T2DM had 2.5 times higher odds of developing sarcopenia over a 5-year period compared to those without T2DM [11].

3. Evaluation of sarcopenia

The evaluation of sarcopenia involves initially screening individuals with a higher likelihood of having the condition, followed by a diagnostic assessment based on key criteria: reduced muscle strength, decreased muscle mass, and impaired physical function. Mnemonic such as "SARC" can be utilized in the evaluation process (**Figure 1**).

3.1 Screening

SARC-F questionnaire is used to assess sarcopenia risk, as recommended by European Working Group on Sarcopenia in the Elderly. SARC-F is a rapid and simple screening method for sarcopenia in the elderly. The SARC-F is a quick five-question checklist that includes strength, assisted walking, rising from a chair, climbing stairs, and falling [12]. In the SARC-F questionnaire, each question is scored from 0 to 2 points, with a total score ranging from a minimum of 0 to a maximum of 10. A sarcopenia risk is present if the sum of the scores for each of the five items is greater than or equal to 4 points. However, it demonstrates high specificity but low sensitivity. In a meta-analysis including 20 studies evaluating screening accuracy revealed the sensitivity of SARC-F ranged from 27% to 39%, the specificity ranged from 63% to 91% [13]. Hence, if this questionnaire is used, many cases of sarcopenia may likely to be missed. The SARC-Calf tool was developed to tackle the challenge of improving sensitivity in assessing sarcopenia. Calf circumference <33 cm in male and <32 cm in female is being used as a cut-off for diagnosis of sarcopenia [14]. It is

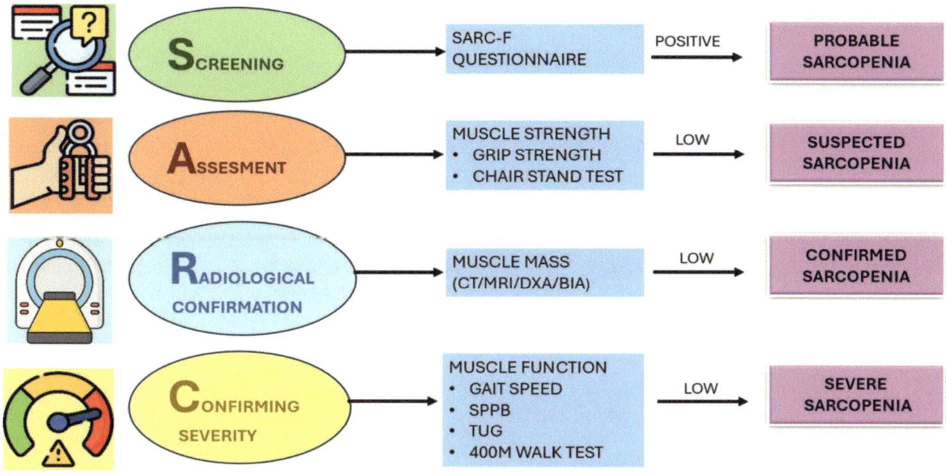

Figure 1.
Evaluation process for sarcopenia [SPPB: short physical performance battery, chair stand test (5 rises), TUG: timed-up and go test].

also recommended to adjust the specified measurements by adding or subtracting a certain number of centimeters based on the patient's body mass index [14].

3.2 Diagnosis

The diagnosis of sarcopenia is based on the presence of low muscle strength, low muscle mass, and poor physical function. Low muscle strength indicates probable sarcopenia, low muscle mass confirms sarcopenia, and poor physical function suggests the severity of sarcopenia. International working groups have set various threshold values for the tests used to evaluate muscle strength, muscle mass, and physical performance in order to define sarcopenia (**Table 1**).

3.2.1 Muscle strength and physical function assessment

Grip strength: Muscle strength is the main parameter for diagnosing sarcopenia. Grip strength moderately correlates with strength in other body compartments. Grip strength in the upper limbs is typically assessed using a manual ergometer. The Jamar® dynamometer, which is validated and widely utilized, is a standard tool for this measurement. Research has indicated that reduced grip strength is associated with unfavorable patient outcomes, including extended hospital stays, increased functional impairments, diminished quality of life, and higher mortality rates [16]. Additionally, diminished hand grip strength is associated with reduced nutritional status and considered a predictive marker of mortality and morbidity [17].

Chair stand test: The test refers to the duration it takes for an individual to rise from a seated position and return to sitting five times consecutively, without using their arms for assistance. If it takes more than 15 seconds for 5 times rising, then it is considered abnormal. Other commonly used tests to assess physical changes include the timed-up and go (TUG) test, where a value of 20 seconds or more indicates impairment; the gait speed (GS) test, with a speed of 0.8 m/second or less; the 400-m walk test, which is considered abnormal if it takes 6 minutes or more or cannot be completed; and the short physical performance battery (SPPB), with a score of

	Low muscle strength	Low muscle mass	Poor physical performance
Revised EWGSOP	*GS*: <27 kg (male) and <16 kg (female) *Chair stand time*: >15 seconds (5 rises)	*ALM*: <20 kg (male) and <15 kg (female) *ALM/height^2*: <7.0 kg/m^2 (male) and <5.5 kg/m^2 (female)	*Gait speed*: 0.8 m/second (4 m course) *SPPB score*: <8 points *TUG*: >20 seconds *400 m walk*: ≥6 minutes or non-completion
Revised AWGS	*GS*: <28 kg (male) and <18 kg (female)	*ALM/height^2*: <7.0 kg/m^2 (male) and <5.4 kg/m^2 (female)	*Gait speed*: <1 m/second (6 m course) *SPPB score*: ≤9 points *Chair stand time*: ≥12 seconds (5 rises)
SDOC	*GS*: <35.5 kg (male) and <20 kg (female) *GS/BMI*: <1.05 kg/body wt (kg)/height (m^2) (male) and <0.79 kg/body wt (kg)/height (m^2) (female) *GS/TBF*: <1.66 kg/TBF (kg) (male) and <0.65 kg/TBF (kg) (female) *GS/arm lean mass*: <6.08 kg/arm lean mass (kg) (male) and <3.26 kg/arm lean mass (kg) (female) *GS/body weight*: <0.45 kg/body wt (kg) (male) and <0.34 kg/body wt (kg) (female)		*Gait speed*: ≤0.8 m/second

Table 1.
Current definition of sarcopenia by various international working groups. EWGSOP: European Working Group on Sarcopenia in Older People; AWGS, Asian Working Group for Sarcopenia; SDOC: Sarcopenia Definitions and Outcomes Consortium; GS: grip strength; ALM: appendicular lean mass; SPPB: short physical performance battery; TUG: timed up-and-go; BMI: body mass index; TBF: total body fat. Adapted from Mesinovic et al. [15].

8 points or less. The latter three tests are particularly useful for grading the severity of sarcopenia [18]. If muscle strength falls below the aforementioned cutoff determined by dynamometry and/or the TUG test, the patient will be classified as having probable sarcopenia, prompting an evaluation of muscle mass.

3.2.2 Muscle mass assessment

Muscle mass refers to the total amount of skeletal muscle in the body. Common techniques for measuring skeletal muscle mass include computed tomography (CT), magnetic resonance imaging (MRI), dual-energy X-ray absorptiometry (DXA), and bioelectrical impedance analysis (BIA). CT and MRI are the current gold standard for assessing muscle mass with high accuracy and reproducibility. CT imaging offers accurate assessments of skeletal muscle mass, commonly using metrics such as skeletal muscle area (SMA), skeletal muscle index (SMI), and muscle radiation attenuation (MRA), which quantifies fat infiltration within the muscle tissue [19]. However, the use of CT imaging is limited due to its high cost and significant radiation exposure. In contrast, DXA is regarded as one of the optimal methods for assessing muscle mass because of its rapid procedure and low radiation exposure.

DXA provides precise analyses of body composition, including bone mineral density (BMD) and distribution between lean and fat masses [19]. Appendicular lean mass (ALM), obtained through DXA scans, represents the sum of the lean mass in the arms and legs. It is commonly used on its own or normalized to height squared (ALM/height^2) or body mass index (ALM/BMI) as an estimate of muscle mass. When appendicular lean mass is divided by height squared (ALM/height^2), it is referred to as the skeletal muscle mass index (SMI). Currently SMI is the most commonly used measure to assess sarcopenia. The BIA is a non-invasive, cheap, easy, and fast method to evaluate body composition without any radiation exposure. BIA is well-suited for large-scale hospital and community screenings due to its simplicity, portability, and affordability, making it a cost-effective alternative for assessing muscle mass.

4. Shared risk factors for development of sarcopenia and diabetes

4.1 Intrinsic risk factors

Aging is one of the most important risk factors for development of diabetes and sarcopenia (**Figure 2**). Beyond the third decade of life, there is gradual loss of skeletal muscle mass and function [20]. The skeletal muscle possesses glucose transporter 4 (GLUT4) responsible for approximately 80% of glucose clearance [21]. Thus, reduced GLUT4, increases susceptibility to T2DM. Age influences muscle health not only by deteriorating its quality and function but also by triggering conditions such as hormone irregularities, mitochondrial impairment, and sustained inflammation, which contribute to sarcopenia. Within muscle fibers, aging leads to changes in DNA and a decline in contractile proteins. Additionally, aging reduces blood flow to muscles, resulting in fewer capillaries and reduced contact between capillaries and muscle fibers, which diminishes the muscle's strength potential. Age-related fibrosis, worsened by elevated oxidative stress and collagen crosslinking, further contributes to increased tissue stiffness [22]. Hormonal imbalances, such as the gradual decline in testosterone levels that occurs as men age, increase the likelihood of developing sarcopenia, as low testosterone is linked to a reduction in muscle mass and strength. Reduced total testosterone levels

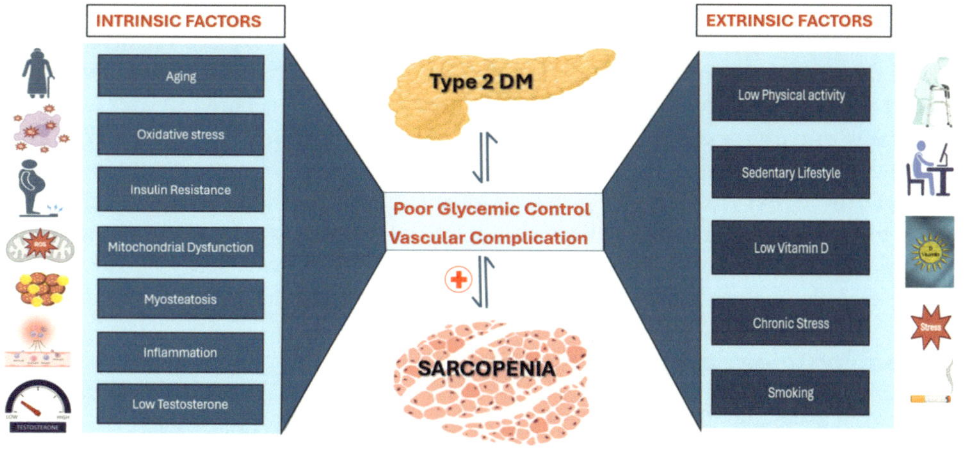

Figure 2.
Shared risk factors and pathophysiology of sarcopenia and type 2 diabetes mellitus.

have been linked to insulin resistance, which increases the likelihood of developing T2DM. Increased production of reactive oxygen species (ROS) disrupts several intracellular signaling pathways, contributing to insulin resistance and impaired β-cell function. Oxidative stress, a key driver of diabetes, plays a central role in its progression. Skeletal muscle ages, reactive oxygen species (ROS) levels gradually rise. Excessive ROS can damage mitochondria, leading to impaired mitochondrial function and possibly contributing to the progression of sarcopenia [23, 24]. Loss of muscle mass and strength is linked to elevated levels of inflammatory markers in the blood, which negatively impact lower limb function and physical activity [25]. Increasing evidence suggests that inflammatory markers are involved in the development and progression of type 2 diabetes. Evidence underscores the crucial role of inflammatory markers in the development of type 2 diabetes. Similarly, sarcopenia is linked to heightened levels of proinflammatory cytokines, such as interleukin 6 (IL-6), tumor necrosis factor-α (TNF-α), and C-reactive protein (CRP). Factors associated with diabetes, such as elevated glycosylated hemoglobin (HbA1c) and the presence of vascular complications, have been linked to an increased likelihood of sarcopenia, with odds ratios of 1.2-fold and 2.4-fold, respectively [26].

4.2 Extrinsic risk factors

A lack of exercise results in insufficient muscle stimulation, reduced protein synthesis, and a gradual decrease in muscle mass (**Figure 2**). Moreover, elderly individuals with a prolonged history of a sedentary lifestyle face a significantly higher risk of developing sarcopenia [27]. Even among older adults who are physically active, sitting for extended periods exceeding 2 hours raises the risk of developing sarcopenia [28]. This underscores the fact that regular exercise alone is not enough to completely offset the harmful effects of prolonged inactivity. Vitamin D is essential for various functions in skeletal muscle, including maintaining muscle excitability by regulating intracellular calcium levels and supporting the proliferation and differentiation of skeletal muscle stem cells [29]. Low levels of vitamin D are linked to reduced physical performance. Studies have shown that vitamin D supplementation can enhance muscle strength and help prevent the atrophy of type II muscle fibers in individuals with vitamin D deficiency [30]. Smokers have higher risk developing T2DM by 30–40%. Various studies have highlighted the harmful effects of smoking on skeletal muscle function and structure, including reduced muscle fatigue resistance due to impaired oxidative capacity and a shift from slow-twitch to fast-twitch muscle fiber types [31, 32]. We investigated the risk factors for sarcopenia in individuals with T2DM, and we identified low BMI, reduced physical activity, hypertension, neuropathy, and low serum calcium levels as significant contributors to the development of sarcopenia in this population [33]. In a study involving 334 hospitalized patients, low BMI, along with lower serum levels of 25(OH)D and IGF-1 (insulin-like growth factor 1), were identified as significant risk factors for sarcopenia in individuals with T2DM [34]. Other factors like chronic stress, and prolonged periods of sleep, can also elevate the risk of muscle loss [35, 36].

5. Pathophysiology of sarcopenia in type 2 DM

As noted earlier, the prevalence of sarcopenia among individuals with T2DM is almost doubled. This is primarily because of overlap of pathophysiologic pathways of both sarcopenia and T2DM. Insulin resistance, oxidative stress, and inflammatory reaction lead to both T2DM and sarcopenia (**Figure 2**).

5.1 Insulin resistance

Insulin resistance, the primary pathophysiological mechanism underlying T2DM, also plays a significant role in the onset and progression of sarcopenia. Skeletal muscle is one of the target organs for insulin action and insulin resistance [37]. Insulin has anabolic effect on skeletal muscle, which gradually decline due to the reduced insulin sensitivity in T2DM. So, the decrease in insulin's effect lead not only to decreased protein synthesis but also to increased protein degradation [38]. Insulin itself reduces proteasome catalytic activity in muscles [39], thus resulting in reductions in muscle mass and strength. There are multiple pathways through which insulin resistance contributes to the development of muscle atrophy. In insulin resistance (IR), elevated blood glucose levels can lead to muscle atrophy through the proteolytic ubiquitin-proteasome pathway [40]. Additionally, metabolic dysregulation caused by IR promotes hyperglycemia and muscle atrophy via the WWP1/KLF15 pathway [41]. WWP1 is a member of the ubiquitin ligase protein family. KLF15 is a protein associated with muscle wasting. Animal studies have shown that hyperglycemia upregulates KLF15 protein in skeletal muscle by downregulating the E3 ubiquitin ligase WWP1, followed by inhibition of ubiquitin-dependent degradation of KLF15. Muscle protein synthesis is mainly regulated by two factors: insulin-like growth factor 1 (IGF1) and myostatin [42]. Myostatin, a member of the transforming growth factor β (TGF-β) superfamily, inhibits mTORC1 signaling and increases AMPKα2 phosphorylation. These processes contribute to the dysregulation of protein synthesis and promote autophagic proteolysis, leading to muscle degradation [43]. Hyperinsulinemia caused by IR increases the content of myostatin, thereby reducing skeletal muscle through the above-mentioned pathway.

5.2 Inflammation

T2DM is characterized by state of chronic low-grade inflammation. Inflammatory markers like IL-6, TNF- , and CRP are commonly elevated in people with T2DM. Higher levels of these pro-inflammatory factors have also been linked to negative effects on muscle mass and function [44]. IL-6 is linked to greater muscle and strength loss in individuals with T2DM, likely due to its direct impact on muscle cells and indirect effects on neurons and blood vessels. The inflammatory cascade starts with the activation of other interleukins, such as TNF and IL-1, which trigger signaling pathways like NFκB and FOXO4, ultimately leading to muscle atrophy [45].

5.3 Oxidative stress

Muscle cells naturally generate reactive oxygen species (ROS), such as hydroxyl radicals, peroxides, and superoxides, as by-products of normal metabolism, making them particularly vulnerable to oxidative stress. In T2DM, hyperglycemia increases ROS production, which activates the ubiquitin-proteasome system, speeding up muscle protein breakdown and contributing to sarcopenia [46]. Studies in diabetic rat have demonstrated that elevated oxidative stress disrupts muscle repair, hinders satellite cell differentiation, and damages DNA [47]. Mitochondria play an important role in muscle function and metabolism. Mitochondrial dysfunction, a factor linked to both aging and T2DM, contributes to oxidative stress and the decline of metabolic and muscle health [48]. In the elderly, oxidative capacity per muscle unit is reduced by 50% compared to younger individuals and is accompanied by a higher incidence of mitochondrial DNA mutations [49]. Mitochondrial dysfunction caused by diabetes promotes myocyte apoptosis, which increases the risk of developing sarcopenia.

5.4 Advanced glycation end products

Hyperglycemia promotes the formation of advanced glycation end products (AGEs), which accumulate in muscle tissue and contribute to the decline in muscle performance [50]. In diabetes, the accumulation AGEs negatively impacts skeletal muscle health by triggering pathways such as mitochondrial dysfunction and cell death. AGEs also disrupt muscle contractility by altering charge properties and increasing intramuscular protein cross-linking. Additionally, AGEs bind to their receptors (RAGE) on skeletal muscle cell membranes, initiating inflammation and activating NADPH oxidase through intracellular signaling. This process elevates circulating reactive oxygen species, exacerbating oxidative stress [51].

5.5 Myosteatosis

Myosteatosis refers to the abnormal accumulation of fat within skeletal muscle. This includes intermuscular adipose tissue (IMAT), intramuscular adipose tissue, and intramyocellular lipids (IMCLs) within muscle cells [52]. Myosteatosis increases with aging and is known to have a negative correlation with muscle mass, strength, and mobility. IMAT is also positively linked to insulin resistance and a higher risk of developing T2DM [53]. However, the precise mechanisms linking intermuscular adipose tissue (IMAT) to insulin resistance and explaining this relationship remain unclear.

6. Holistic approaches to managing sarcopenia in type 2 diabetes mellitus

The primary goals of treating sarcopenia are to reverse or stabilize the loss of muscle strength or to some extent increasing lean muscle mass, thus improving quality of life and the ability to perform daily activities. Currently, there are limited management options available for treating sarcopenia. At present, nutritional intervention and physical activity are considered the most promising strategies for addressing sarcopenia.

6.1 Nutritional intervention

Proper nutritional intervention plays a critical role in managing sarcopenia in individuals with diabetes. Nutritional interventions have the ability to prevent or potentially reverse sarcopenia and frailty by supporting muscle maintenance and improving overall physical health. The majority of studies have consistently demonstrated the beneficial effects of dietary and nutritional interventions in preventing and managing sarcopenia [54–56]. A balanced diet rich in high-quality protein, essential amino acids (particularly leucine), vitamins, and minerals is crucial for stimulating muscle protein synthesis and preventing muscle loss.

6.1.1 Protein

Boosting protein intake can significantly enhance blood sugar regulation, support muscle preservation, aid in weight management, lower inflammation, and improve insulin sensitivity. Increase in protein consumption has been shown to improve grip strength and reduce occurrence of sarcopenia [57]. Research has indicated that older adults with sarcopenia should consume 1.6 g of protein per kg of body weight daily. Similarly, the ESPEN expert group and the PROT-AGE study group recommend a daily protein intake of approximately 1.2–1.5 g per kg of body weight for individuals with chronic conditions like diabetes [58, 59]. Animal protein intake has been associated with a higher overall risk of developing T2DM compared to plant protein intake [60]. Therefore, protein derived from plant may be the most appropriate source to ensure protein needs in older adults with or at risk of T2DM. Essential amino acids are crucial for both muscle building and maintenance. A recent prospective study of 1140 T2DM patients revealed that the higher baseline levels of branched-chain amino acids valine, leucine, and isoleucine significantly lower the risk of muscle mass loss over time [61]. Long-term consumption of leucine-enriched essential amino acids, when combined with exercise, has a synergistic effect on increasing skeletal muscle mass, strength, and walking speed in elderly individuals [62]. This combination can be an effective countermeasure to sarcopenia. As a result, supplementation with branched-chain amino acids, especially leucine or leucine-rich proteins, is among the most commonly used strategies for managing sarcopenia in older adults.

6.1.2 Omega-3 fatty acids

Omega-3 fatty acids have shown potential benefits in the prevention and management of sarcopenia. Omega-3 fatty acids may support muscle health by promoting protein synthesis, improving muscle mass, and enhancing muscle strength. Omega-3 fatty acid supplementation affects muscle directly by increasing muscle protein synthesis [63]. A meta-analysis of 66 randomized controlled trials investigating omega-3 long-chain polyunsaturated fatty acids as an intervention for muscle-related outcomes found that omega-3 supplementation had positive effects on certain measures, such as skeletal muscle mass and quadricep strength. However, other outcomes, including mid-arm muscle circumference and hand grip strength, remained unaffected [64]. Additionally, their anti-inflammatory properties can help reduce chronic low-grade inflammation, which is often associated with sarcopenia and conditions like type 2 diabetes. A meta-regression analysis of 45 randomized controlled trials found that omega-3 fatty acid supplementation significantly improved HbA1c levels in individuals with T2DM. However, it showed no significant changes in other glycemic markers, such as fasting glucose, insulin levels, and HOMA-IR [65].

6.1.3 Vitamin D

Vitamin D has been shown to enhance muscle mass and function, making it beneficial for patients with sarcopenia. However, data on sarcopenia on vitamin D supplementation has been conflicting. Meta-analyses have shown positive effects of supplementation, but these benefits are primarily observed in individuals with 25-hydroxyvitamin D levels below 25 or 30 nmol/L [66]. However, two recent meta-analyses have reported either no significant impact or even negative effects on physical performance, including measures such as the short physical performance battery scores and timed up-and-go tests [67, 68]. One study demonstrated that combining exercise with daily supplementation of whey protein (22 g), essential amino acids (11 g, including 4 g of leucine), and vitamin D (100 IU) led to an increase in lean mass nearly 2 kg greater than exercise alone in older adults with sarcopenia [69]. Moreover, the combination treatment significantly improved hand grip strength and reduced CRP levels, indicating enhanced muscle function and decreased inflammation. As a result, adequate vitamin D intake is recommended for elderly diabetic individuals, particularly those with sarcopenia. However, the ideal dose, frequency, and duration of vitamin D supplementation remain uncertain.

6.2 Physical exercise

Physical exercise is regarded as an effective intervention for preventing and managing diabetes mellitus associated with sarcopenia. Both aerobic and resistance exercises are effective in preventing and managing the loss of muscle mass and strength associated with aging. Aerobic exercise improves glycemic parameters by reducing HbA1c levels, fasting blood glucose, and insulin resistance and also enhances skeletal muscle mass, especially improving leg strength. Resistance exercise strengthens muscles, improves insulin sensitivity, reduces fat accumulation, and preserves mitochondrial function in individuals with T2DM [70]. Resistance training is widely recognized as an effective approach for enhancing muscle mass and function in older adults with sarcopenia and is considered the primary treatment for this condition. A meta-analysis of 26 trials examined the effects of different exercise modes on various aspects of sarcopenia in older adults. The results showed that resistance exercise, as well as combined resistance and aerobic exercise, led to improvements in knee extension strength, gait speed, and timed up and go (TUG) performance [71]. Resistance training, when combined with nutritional supplements, can enhance its effectiveness as an intervention. International guidelines recommend that individuals with T2DM engage in resistance training at least twice per week [72]. Older adults with chronic conditions to engage in 150 to 300 minutes of moderate to vigorous-intensity physical activity (MVPA) per week and to minimize sedentary behavior, as recommended by World Health Organization [73]. A recent meta-analysis in older adults (n = 43,796) showed that higher total physical activity levels and avoiding sedentary behavior were associated with better upper and lower body muscle strength, as well as improved upper and lower body muscle power [74]. However, compensatory increases in sedentary behavior may diminish or negate the metabolic and muscle health benefits of physical activity interventions. To counteract the harmful effects of sitting for more than 8 hours a day on all-cause mortality, high levels of moderate to vigorous physical activity (60–75 minutes per day) are necessary [75]. The Tromsø study, conducted on 3653 community-dwelling individuals, found that older adults who engage in moderate levels of MVPA have lower chances of developing probable sarcopenia, even if they spend a significant amount of time being sedentary [76]. The evidence from interventions aimed specifically at reducing sedentary behavior remains inconclusive. Growing evidences indicate that both engaging in more MVPA and reducing sedentary behavior contribute to improved metabolic and muscle health in older adults. Notably, for older adults and patients with neurological conditions, high-intensity exercise can be challenging to perform. However, blood flow restriction (BFR) training offers a viable alternative to traditional exercise, as even low-intensity strength training with BFR can lead to significant improvements in muscle strength [77].

6.3 Pharmacotherapy

At present, there are no approved medications specifically for the treatment of sarcopenia. However, several drugs have demonstrated promising efficacy in recent clinical trials. Myostatin-based medications have generated significant interest due to their potential to enhance muscle growth and counteract muscle loss. Myostatin is a cytokine known as growth and differentiation factor-8 (GDF-8), primarily produced and secreted by skeletal muscles. It serves as a negative regulator of muscle mass. In simple terms, myostatin binds to the activin receptor type IIB (ActRIIB), triggering the activation of SMAD2/3, which in turn suppresses the expression of MyoD. MyoD is crucial for the differentiation and repair of skeletal muscle. Myostatin inhibitors, such as propeptides, soluble receptors, antibodies, and natural antagonists, have been tested in clinical trials to assess their ability to improve muscle growth and strength. However, despite showing potential for increasing muscle mass, these myostatin inhibitors have shown limited or no benefits in improving physical function, which is a more clinically important outcome for patients. Androgens play a crucial role in the development and maintenance of skeletal muscle [78]. Due to their anabolic effects on muscle tissue, they are considered highly promising for the treatment of sarcopenia. Testosterone treatment has been shown to be effective in increasing muscle mass and, to a lesser extent, improving muscle strength. However, similar to myostatin-based agonists, the evidence supporting the beneficial effects of testosterone treatment on physical performance in older adults is inconsistent. Adverse side effects of testosterone treatment, such as transaminitis, benign prostatic hypertrophy, and uterine hyperproliferation, limit its widespread use, especially in older adults. These potential risks must be carefully considered when evaluating testosterone as a treatment for sarcopenia. Selective androgen receptor modulators (SARMs) are designed to promote muscle growth and improve bone health while reducing unwanted side effects on other tissues, such as the prostate. In a randomized placebo-controlled study of 170 sarcopenic frail women, MK-0773, a selective androgen receptor modulator (SARM), was administered. The results showed a statistically significant increase in lean body mass (LBM) from baseline at month 6 compared to the placebo. However, this increase in muscle mass did not translate into improvements in strength or physical function [79]. Increasing muscle mass through pharmacological treatments alone provides limited functional benefits. Therefore, incorporating targeted exercise, particularly resistance training, will likely be crucial for achieving improvements in physical function in future clinical trials.

6.3.1 Antidiabetic drug

As previously mentioned, hyperglycemia leads to reduced mitochondrial activity, heightened oxidative stress, and increased inflammation, all of which contribute to insulin resistance and muscle atrophy by disrupting insulin signaling pathways. For individuals with diabetes and sarcopenia, managing blood sugar levels is crucial. Keeping blood glucose under control can help reduce muscle loss and limit protein breakdown. In individuals with well-managed diabetes, stable insulin levels support muscle protein synthesis, improving muscle quality and strength. This not only helps prevent sarcopenia but also supports muscle growth and repair, improving overall muscle health and physical performance. Multiple antidiabetic drugs are used to manage hyperglycemia, but each medication has a varying impact on muscle mass and muscle strength.

While antidiabetic drugs may influence muscle mass, the exact mechanisms of most of these medications on sarcopenia remain unclear. Metformin, a commonly used drug for treating T2DM, has shown positive effects on muscle mass and muscle strength in various studies [80, 81]. Some antidiabetic drugs, especially sulfonylureas like glinide, gliclazide, and glibenclamide, have been linked to muscle loss or injury. These drugs work by inhibiting the KATP channels, which in turn stimulates insulin secretion, but their long-term use may have negative effects on muscle tissue. Thiazolidinediones act as insulin sensitizers. Insulin resistance is one of the pathophysiological mechanisms for development of sarcopenia, so these may be beneficial for muscle performance in diabetics. Improvement in insulin resistance promotes favorable changes in PI3K/Akt signaling and reduces activation of caspase-3 pathways, ultimately leading to a decrease in proteolysis and muscle shrinkage [82]. Pioglitazone, in particular, boosts skeletal muscle energy use by lowering fat accumulation within muscles and enhancing fatty acid metabolism [83]. Dipeptidyl peptidase-4 inhibitors (DPP-4) have shown to have positive effects on muscle mass [84]. A small study involving 80 elderly diabetic patients found that treatment with DPP-4 inhibitors was associated with improved sarcopenic parameters, including fat-free mass, skeletal muscle mass, muscle strength, and gait speed [85]. Glucagon-like peptide 1 receptor agonists (GLP-1RAs) possess anti-inflammatory and antioxidant properties, though their exact mechanism of action on skeletal muscle remains a topic of ongoing research and discussion. Animal studies have shown sodium-glucose cotransporter 2 inhibitors (SGLT-2i) enhanced fatty acid metabolism in muscles, helping to prevent muscle wasting [86]. Despite the potential benefits suggested by preclinical studies, the effects of SGLT-2i on muscle remain uncertain due to the limited follow-up periods in clinical trials. Insulin therapy is associated with weight gain, which could be beneficial for patients with a low BMI. A population-based KORA-Age study found that insulin therapy was linked to an increase in skeletal muscle index, but it showed no association with improvements in grip strength or performance on the timed up and go (TUG) test [87]. However, limited studies indicate that long-term insulin use may negatively impact muscle health. Consequently, there is no consistent evidence to support the use of insulin therapy for managing sarcopenia in older adults.

7. Conclusion

Type 2 diabetes mellitus and sarcopenia share a bidirectional relationship. Overlapping pathophysiological mechanisms, such as insulin resistance, inflammation, oxidative stress, accumulation of advanced glycation end products (AGEs), myosteatosis, and the aging process itself contribute to the development of both conditions. Currently, there are no approved targeted therapies for the management of sarcopenia. A few treatments, such as myostatin antagonists, testosterone supplementation, and selective androgen receptor modulators have been explored, but many remain in the experimental or clinical trial stages. The mainstay of management involves dietary adjustments emphasizing foods rich in protein, essential amino acids, vitamin D, calcium, and other vital nutrients such as omega-3 fatty acids. Additionally, incorporating regular physical activity, particularly resistance exercises, and minimizing sedentary behavior are key components. A wide range of antidiabetic medications is available for glycemic control, each with potential positive or negative effects on muscle mass and function. Therefore, selecting the appropriate diabetic medication is crucial when managing sarcopenia.

Author details

Jaya Bhanu Kanwar
Department of Endocrinology, IMS and SUM Hospital, Bhubaneswar, Odisha, India

*Address all correspondence to: jbk.endo@gmail.com

References

[1] Sayer AA, Cooper R, Arai H, Cawthon PM, Ntsama Essomba MJ, Fielding RA, et al. Sarcopenia. Nature Reviews. Disease Primers. 2024;**10**(1):68

[2] Filippin LI, de Oliveira Teixeira VN, da Silva MPM, Miraglia F, da Silva FS. Sarcopenia: A predictor of mortality and the need for early diagnosis and intervention. Aging Clinical and Experimental Research. 2015;**27**(3):249-254

[3] Yeung SS, Reijnierse EM, Pham VK, Trappenburg MC, Lim WK, Meskers CG, et al. Sarcopenia and its association with falls and fractures in older adults: A systematic review and meta-analysis. Journal of Cachexia, Sarcopenia and Muscle. 2019;**10**:485-500

[4] Cawthon PM, Manini T, Patel SM, Newman A, Travison T, Kiel DP, et al. Putative cut-points in sarcopenia components and incident adverse health outcomes: An SDOC analysis. Journal of the American Geriatrics Society. 2020;**68**:1429-1437

[5] Anker SD et al. Welcome to the ICD-10 code for sarcopenia. Journal of Cachexia, Sarcopenia and Muscle. 2016;**7**:512-514

[6] Egan B, Zierath JR. Exercise metabolism and the molecular regulation of skeletal muscle adaptation. Cell Metabolism. 2013;**17**(2):162-184

[7] Compston J. Type 2 diabetes mellitus and bone. Journal of Internal Medicine. 2018;**283**(2):140-153

[8] Petermann-Rocha F, Balntzi V, Gray SR, Lara J, Ho FK, Pell JP, et al. Global prevalence of sarcopenia and severe sarcopenia: A systematic review and meta-analysis. Journal of Cachexia, Sarcopenia and Muscle. 2022;**13**:86-99

[9] Dai S, Shu D, Meng F, Chen Y, Wang J, Liu X, et al. Higher risk of sarcopenia in older adults with type 2 diabetes: NHANES 1999-2018. Obesity Facts. 2023;**16**:237-248

[10] Das S. The impact of diabetes on sarcopenia in community-dwelling older adults in India: Key findings from the longitudinal ageing study in India (LASI). Diabetes Epidemiology and Management. 2023;**12**:100158

[11] Nakamura K, Yoshida D, Honda T, Hata J, Shibata M, Hirakawa Y, et al. Midlife and late-life diabetes and sarcopenia in a general older Japanese population: The Hisayama Study. Journal of Diabetes Investigation. 2021;**12**:1899-1907

[12] Malmstrom TK, Morley JE. SARC-F: A simple questionnaire to rapidly diagnose sarcopenia. Journal of the American Medical Directors Association. 2013;**14**(8):531-532

[13] Lu J-L, Ding L-Y, Xu Q, Zhu S, Xu X-Y, Hua H-X, et al. Screening accuracy of SARC-F for Sarcopenia in the elderly: A diagnostic meta-analysis. The Journal of Nutrition, Health & Aging. 2021;**25**:172-182

[14] Gonzalez MC, Mehrnezhad A, Razaviarab N, Barbosa-Silva TG, Heymsfield SB. Calf circumference: Cutoff values from the NHANES 1999-2006. The American Journal of Clinical Nutrition. 2021;**113**(6):1679-1687

[15] Mesinovic J, Fyfe JJ, Talevski J, et al. Type 2 diabetes mellitus and sarcopenia as comorbid chronic diseases in older

adults: Established and emerging treatments and therapies. Diabetes & Metabolism Journal. 2023;**47**(6):719-742

[16] Leong DP, Teo KK, Rangarajan S, Lopez-Jaramillo P, Avezum A, Orlandini A, et al. Prognostic value of grip strength: Findings from the prospective urban rural epidemiology (PURE) study. Lancet. 2015;**386**:266-273

[17] Cederholm T, Jensen G, Correia MIT, Gonzalez MC, Fukushima R, Higashiguchi T, et al. GLIM criteria for the diagnosis of malnutrition A consensus report from the global clinical nutrition community. Journal of Cachexia, Sarcopenia and Muscle. 2019;**10**(1):207-217

[18] de Luis RD, Gómez JC, García-Almeida JM, Vallo FG, Rolo GG, Gómez JJL, et al. Diabetic Sarcopenia. A proposed muscle screening protocol in people with diabetes: Expert document. Reviews in Endocrine & Metabolic Disorders. 2024;**25**(4):651-661

[19] Ackermans LLGC, Rabou J, Basrai M, Schweinlin A, Bischoff SC, Cussenot O, et al. Screening, diagnosis and monitoring of sarcopenia: When to use which tool? Clinical Nutrition ESPEN. 2022;**48**:36-44

[20] Volpi E, Nazemi R, Fujita S. Muscle tissue changes with aging. Current Opinion in Clinical Nutrition and Metabolic Care. 2004;**7**(4):405-410

[21] Son JW, Lee SS, Kim SR, et al. Low muscle mass and risk of type 2 diabetes in middle-aged and older adults: Findings from the KoGES. Diabetologia. 2017;**60**(5):865-872

[22] Granic A et al. Hallmarks of ageing in human skeletal muscle and implications for understanding the pathophysiology of sarcopenia in women and men. Clinical Science. 2023;**137**:1721-1751

[23] Fealy CE, Grevendonk L, Hoeks J, Hesselink MKC. Skeletal muscle mitochondrial network dynamics in metabolic disorders and aging. Trends in Molecular Medicine. 2021;**27**(11):1033-1044

[24] Gonzalez-Freire M, Scalzo P, D'Agostino J, Moore ZA, Diaz-Ruiz A, Fabbri E, et al. Skeletal muscle ex vivo mitochondrial respiration parallels decline in vivo oxidative capacity, cardiorespiratory fitness, and muscle strength: The Baltimore Longitudinal Study of Aging. Aging Cell. 2018;**17**(2):e12725

[25] Suzuki K. Chronic inflammation as an immunological abnormality and effectiveness of exercise. Biomolecules. 2019;**9**(6):223

[26] Feng L, Gao Q, Hu K, Wu M, Wang Z, Chen F, et al. Prevalence and risk factors of sarcopenia in patients with diabetes: A metaanalysis. The Journal of Clinical Endocrinology and Metabolism. 2022;**107**:1470-1483

[27] Giallauria F, Cittadini A, Smart NA, Vigorito C. Resistance training and sarcopenia. Monaldi Archives for Chest Disease. 2016;**84**(1-2):738

[28] de Souza LF, Danielewicz AL, Rech CR, d'Orsi E, Mendonça VA, Lacerda ACR, et al. How much time in sedentary behavior is associated with probable sarcopenia in older adults? Geriatric Nursing. 2022;**48**:127-131

[29] Uchitomi R, Oyabu M, Kamei Y. Vitamin D and sarcopenia: Potential of vitamin D supplementation in sarcopenia prevention and treatment. Nutrients. 2020;**12**(10):3189

[30] Kalyani RR, Metter EJ, Egan J, et al. Hyperglycemia predicts persistently lower muscle strength with aging. Diabetes Care. 2015;**38**(1):82-90

[31] Degens H, Veerkamp JH. Changes in oxidative capacity and fatigue resistance in skeletal muscle. The International Journal of Biochemistry. 1994;**26**(7):871-878

[32] Orlander J, Kiessling KH, Larsson L. Skeletal muscle metabolism, morphology and function in sedentary smokers and nonsmokers. Acta Physiologica Scandinavica. 1979;**107**(1):39-46

[33] Sravya SL, Swain J, Sahoo AK, Mangaraj S, Kanwar J, Jadhao P, et al. Sarcopenia in type 2 diabetes mellitus: Study of the modifiable risk factors involved. Journal of Clinical Medicine. 2023;**12**(17):5499

[34] Du Y, Wang Y, Zhang P, Zhong X, Pan T. Analysis of risk factors for the association of sarcopenia in patients with type 2 diabetes mellitus. Diabetes, Metabolic Syndrome and Obesity. 2024;**17**:1455-1466

[35] Stefanaki C, Pervanidou P, Boschiero D, Chrousos GP. Chronic stress and body composition disorders: Implications for health and disease. Hormones. 2018;**17**(1):33-43

[36] Li X, He J, Sun Q. Sleep duration and sarcopenia: An updated systematic review and meta-analysis. Journal of the American Medical Directors Association. 2023;**24**(8):1193-206.e5

[37] Yaribeygi H, Farrokhi FR, Butler AE, et al. Insulin resistance: Review of the underlying molecular mechanisms. Journal of Cellular Physiology. 2019;**234**(6):8152-8161

[38] Izzo A, Massimino E, Riccardi G, et al. A narrative review on sarcopenia in type 2 diabetes mellitus: Prevalence and associated factors. Nutrients. 2021;**13**(1):183

[39] Russell ST, Rajani S, Dhadda RS, et al. Mechanism of induction of muscle protein loss by hyperglycaemia. Experimental Cell Research. 2009;**315**(1):16-25

[40] Purnamasari D, Tetrasiwi EN, Kartiko GJ, et al. Sarcopenia and chronic complications of type 2 diabetes mellitus. The Review of Diabetic Studies. 2022;**18**(3):157-165

[41] Mcbride MJ, Foley KP, D'souza DM, et al. The NLRP3 inflammasome contributes to sarcopenia and lower muscle glycolytic potential in old mice. American Journal of Physiology. Endocrinology and Metabolism. 2017;**313**(2):E222-E232

[42] Glass DJ. Skeletal muscle hypertrophy and atrophy signaling pathways. The International Journal of Biochemistry & Cell Biology. 2005;**37**(10):1974-1984

[43] Qiu J, Thapaliya S, Runkana A, et al. Hyperammonemia in cirrhosis induces transcriptional regulation of myostatin by an NF-kappaB-mediated mechanism. Proceedings of the National Academy of Sciences. 2013;**110**(45):18162-18167

[44] Visser M, Pahor M, Taaffe DR, et al. Relationship of interleukin-6 and tumor necrosis factor-alpha with muscle mass and muscle strength in elderly men and women: The health ABC study. The Journals of Gerontology. Series A, Biological Sciences and Medical Sciences. 2002;**57**(5):M326-M332

[45] Giha HA, Alamin OAO, Sater MS. Diabetic sarcopenia: Metabolic and molecular appraisal. Acta Diabetologica. 2022;**59**(8):989-1000

[46] Bowen TS, Schuler G, Adams V. Skeletal muscle wasting in cachexia and sarcopenia: Molecular pathophysiology

and impact of exercise training. Journal of Cachexia, Sarcopenia and Muscle. 2015;**6**(3):197-207

[47] Aragno M, Mastrocola R, Catalano MG, et al. Oxidative stress impairs skeletal muscle repair in diabetic rats. Diabetes. 2004;**53**(4):1082-1088

[48] Short KR, Bigelow ML, Kahl J, et al. Decline in skeletal muscle mitochondrial function with aging in humans. Proceedings of the National Academy of Sciences. 2005;**102**(15):5618-5623

[49] Bua E, Johnson J, Herbst A, et al. Mitochondrial DNA-deletion mutations accumulate intracellularly to detrimental levels in aged human skeletal muscle fibers. American Journal of Human Genetics. 2006;**79**(3):469-480

[50] Hou Y, Xiang J, Wang B, Duan S, Song R, Zhou W, et al. Pathogenesis and comprehensive treatment strategies of sarcopenia in elderly patients with type 2 diabetes mellitus. Frontiers in Endocrinology. 2024;**14**:1263650

[51] Suzuki A, Yabu A, Nakamura H. Advanced glycation end products in musculoskeletal system and disorders. Methods. 2022;**203**:179-186

[52] Correa-de-Araujo R, Addison O, Miljkovic I, Goodpaster BH, Bergman BC, Clark RV, et al. Myosteatosis in the context of skeletal muscle function deficit: An Interdisciplinary Workshop at the National Institute on Aging. Frontiers in Physiology. 2020;**11**:963

[53] Addison O, Marcus RL, Lastayo PC, Ryan AS. Intermuscular fat: A review of the consequences and causes. International Journal of Endocrinology. 2014;**2014**:309570

[54] Henson J, Arsenyadis F, Redman E, Brady EM, Coull NA, Edwardson CL, et al. Relative protein intake and associations with markers of physical function in those with type 2 diabetes. Diabetic Medicine. 2022;**39**(8):e14851

[55] Casals-Vázquez C, Suárez-Cadenas E, Estébanez Carvajal FM, Aguilar Trujillo MP, Jiménez Arcos MM, Vázquez Sáchez M. Relationship between quality of life, physical activity, nutrition, glycemic control and sarcopenia in older adults with type 2 diabetes mellitus. Nutrición Hospitalaria. 2017;**34**(5):1198-1204

[56] Fanelli SM, Kelly OJ, Krok-Schoen JL, Taylor CA. Low protein intakes and poor diet quality associate with functional limitations in US adults with diabetes: A 2005-2016 NHANES analysis. Nutrients. 2021;**13**(8):2582

[57] Wu Y, de Crom TO, Schaft NVD, Chen Z, Rivadeneira F, Boer CG, et al. Dietary protein intake with body composition, hand grip strength, and sarcopenia in older adults: A population-based study. Clinical Nutrition ESPEN. 2023;**54**:476

[58] Deutz NE, Bauer JM, Barazzoni R, Biolo G, Boirie Y, Bosy-Westphal A, et al. Protein intake and exercise for optimal muscle function with aging: Recommendations from the ESPEN Expert Group. Clinical Nutrition. 2014;**33**(6):929-936

[59] Bauer J, Biolo G, Cederholm T, Cesari M, Cruz-Jentoft AJ, Morley JE, et al. Evidence-based recommendations for optimal dietary protein intake in older people: A position paper from the PROT-AGE Study Group. Journal of the American Medical Directors Association. 2013;**14**(8):542-559

[60] Shang X, Scott D, Hodge AM, et al. Dietary protein intake and risk of type 2 diabetes: Results from the Melbourne

Collaborative Cohort Study and a meta-analysis of prospective studies. The American Journal of Clinical Nutrition. 2016;**104**(5):1352-1365

[61] Low S, Wang J, Moh A, et al. Amino acid profile of skeletal muscle loss in type 2 diabetes: Results from a 7-year longitudinal study in asians. Diabetes Research and Clinical Practice. 2022;**186**:109803

[62] Kobayashi H. Amino acid nutrition in the prevention and treatment of sarcopenia. Yakugaku Zasshi. 2018;**138**(10):1277-1283

[63] Smith GI, Atherton P, Reeds DN, et al. Dietary omega-3 fatty acid supplementation increases the rate of muscle protein synthesis in older adults: A randomized controlled trial. The American Journal of Clinical Nutrition. 2011;**93**(2):402-412

[64] Bird JK, Troesch B, Warnke I, Calder PC. The effect of long chain omega-3 polyunsaturated fatty acids on muscle mass and function in sarcopenia: A scoping systematic review and meta-analysis. Clinical Nutrition ESPEN. 2021;**46**:73-86

[65] O'Mahoney LL, Matu J, Price OJ, Birch KM, Ajjan RA, Farrar D, et al. Omega-3 polyunsaturated fatty acids favourably modulate cardiometabolic biomarkers in type 2 diabetes: A metaanalysis and meta-regression of randomized controlled trials. Cardiovascular Diabetology. 2018;**17**:98

[66] Beaudart C, Buckinx F, Rabenda V, Gillain S, Cavalier E, Slomian J, et al. The effects of vitamin D on skeletal muscle strength muscle mass, and muscle power: A systematic review and metaanalysis of randomized controlled trials. The Journal of Clinical Endocrinology and Metabolism. 2014;**99**:4336-4345

[67] Bislev LS, Grove-Laugesen D, Rejnmark L. Vitamin D and muscle health: A systematic review and meta-analysis of randomized placebo-controlled trials. Journal of Bone and Mineral Research. 2021;**36**:1651-1660

[68] Prokopidis K, Giannos P, Katsikas Triantafyllidis K, Kechagias KS, Mesinovic J, Witard OC, et al. Effect of vitamin D monotherapy on indices of sarcopenia in community-dwelling older adults: A systematic review and meta-analysis. Journal of Cachexia, Sarcopenia and Muscle. 2022;**13**:1642-1652

[69] Rondanelli M, Klersy C, Terracol G, Talluri J, Maugeri R, Guido D, et al. Whey protein, amino acids, and vitamin D supplementation with physical activity increases fat-free mass and strength, functionality, and quality of life and decreases inflammation in sarcopenic elderly. The American Journal of Clinical Nutrition. 2016;**103**(3):830-840

[70] Bird SR, Hawley JA. Update on the effects of physical activity on insulin sensitivity in humans. BMJ Open Sport & Exercise Medicine. 2016;**2**(1):e000143

[71] Lu L, Mao L, Feng Y, Ainsworth BE, Liu Y, Chen N. Effects of different exercise training modes on muscle strength and physical performance in older people with sarcopenia: A systematic review and meta-analysis. BMC Geriatrics. 2021;**21**:708

[72] Hordern MD, Dunstan DW, Prins JB, Baker MK, Singh MA, Coombes JS. Exercise prescription for patients with type 2 diabetes and pre-diabetes: A position statement from Exercise and Sport Science Australia. Journal of Science and Medicine in Sport. 2012;**15**(1):25-31

[73] Bull FC, Al-Ansari SS, Biddle S, Borodulin K, Buman MP, Cardon G,

et al. World Health Organization 2020 guidelines on physical activity and sedentary behaviour. British Journal of Sports Medicine. 2020;**54**:1451-1462

[74] Ramsey KA, Rojer AG, D'Andrea L, Otten RH, Heymans MW, Trappenburg MC, et al. The association of objectively measured physical activity and sedentary behavior with skeletal muscle strength and muscle power in older adults: A systematic review and meta-analysis. Ageing Research Reviews. 2021;**67**:101266

[75] Madden KM, Feldman B, Chase J. Sedentary time and metabolic risk in extremely active older adults. Diabetes Care. 2021;**44**:194-200

[76] Johansson J, Morseth B, Scott D, Strand BH, Hopstock LA, Grimsgaard S. Moderate-to-vigorous physical activity modifies the relationship between sedentary time and sarcopenia: The Tromso Study 2015-2016. Journal of Cachexia, Sarcopenia and Muscle. 2021;**12**:955-963

[77] Zhang XZ, Xie WQ, Chen L, et al. Blood flow restriction training for the intervention of sarcopenia: Current stage and future perspective. Frontiers in Medicine. 2022;**9**:894996

[78] Becker C, Lord SR, Studenski SA, Warden SJ, Fielding RA, Recknor CP, et al. Myostatin antibody (LY2495655) in older weak fallers: A proof-of-concept, randomised, phase 2 trial. The Lancet Diabetes and Endocrinology. 2015;**3**:948-957

[79] Papanicolaou DA, Ather SN, Zhu H, Zhou Y, Lutkiewicz J, Scott BB, et al. A phase IIA randomized, placebo-controlled clinical trial to study the efficacy and safety of the selective androgen receptor modulator (SARM), MK-0773 in female participants with sarcopenia. The Journal of Nutrition, Health & Aging. 2013;**17**:533-543

[80] Wu CN, Tien KJ. The impact of antidiabetic agents on sarcopenia in type 2 diabetes: A literature review. Journal Diabetes Research. 2020;**2020**:9368583

[81] Massimino E, Izzo A, Riccardi G, et al. The impact of glucose-lowering drugs on sarcopenia in type 2 diabetes: Current evidence and underlying mechanisms. Cells. 2021;**10**(8):1958

[82] Coletta DK, Sriwijitkamol A, Wajcberg E, Tantiwong P, Li M, Prentki M, et al. Pioglitazone stimulates AMP-activated protein kinase signalling and increases the expression of genes involved in adiponectin signalling, mitochondrial function and fat oxidation in human skeletal muscle in vivo: A randomised trial. Diabetologia. 2009;**52**(4):723-732

[83] Yokota T, Kinugawa S, Hirabayashi K, et al. Pioglitazone improves whole-body aerobic capacity and skeletal muscle energy metabolism in patients with metabolic syndrome. Journal of Diabetes Investigation. 2017;**8**(4):535-541

[84] Sencan C, Dost FS, Ates Bulut E, et al. DPP4 inhibitors as a potential therapeutic option for sarcopenia: A 6-month follow-up study in diabetic older patients. Experimental Gerontology. 2022;**164**:111832

[85] Rizzo MR, Barbieri M, Fava I, Desiderio M, Coppola C, Marfella R, et al. Sarcopenia in elderly diabetic patients: Role of dipeptidyl peptidase 4 inhibitors. Journal of the American Medical Directors Association. 2016;**17**(10):896-901

[86] Bamba R, Okamura T, Hashimoto Y, et al. Extracellular lipidome change by an SGLT2 inhibitor, luseogliflozin,

contributes to prevent skeletal muscle atrophy in db/db mice. Journal of Cachexia, Sarcopenia and Muscle. 2022;**13**(1):574-588

[87] Ferrari U, Then C, Rottenkolber M, Selte C, Seissler J, Conzade R, et al. Longitudinal association of type 2 diabetes and insulin therapy with muscle parameters in the KORA-age study. Acta Diabetologica. 2020;**57**(9):1057-1063